I0608214

Cindy Williams

June 7, 1995

Joyce Morris
16161 Ventura Blvd., Suite 802
Encino, CA 91436

Dear Joyce,

As you know, I believe in Reiki and have used it many times with subtle as well as dramatic results. I think it is so important for the world to understand that healing can occur through one's own hands. Mankind grows closer to God as he comes to this understanding.

I hope that your book, <u>Reiki, Hands That Heal</u>, reaches and gives help to many, many people.

Sincerely,

Cindy Williams

American Chiropractic Associates - Lifestyle Chiropractic   2317 WEST UNIVERSITY DRIVE, SUITE B5
DENTON, TEXAS 76201-1699

AUTO, SPORTS, WORK INJURIES · ACUTE AND CHRONIC PAIN · FAMILY CARE   (817) 387-0405

To the Reiki therapists of tomorrow:

It was a pleasure to review the pre-publication edition of this excellent book. A comprehensive, in depth, text was long overdue. This book is a must for anyone interested in energy medicine.

Reiki is a powerful addition to the toolbox of any health practitioner. Chiropractors, medical doctors, massage therapists and physical therapists all can benefit their patients extraordinarily with Reiki up their sleeves.

Reiki is spreading like wildfire nationwide, and for good reason. It works!

Sincerely,

George Avera, D.C.
Reiki Master Therapist

Susan C. Imbert, NCC, MFCC
Licensed Marriage Family Child Couselor # mfc24772
National Certified Counselor: NCC # 18123
4340 Fulton Avenue, Suite 220
Sherman Oaks, California 91423
818-783-0436

Joyce's book eloquently details the many complexities of Reiki. In keeping with the traditions of the original Reiki Masters, she has compiled this sacred knowledge from Tibetan Sutras into a format anyone understand and use. Photographs illustatrate hand positions. Suggested guidelines recommend which positions might be most effective in what usage. Procedures are appended with information from Traditional Oriental Medicine as well as Western medical constructs.

What makes this book different from others is the sense one gets of the author herself. One can almost feel the empathy and healing energy from the pages, just as one might sense from speaking with her in person. However, the miracle of Reiki can best be comprehended by the experience of it, such as the time she took someone's hand, and severe second degree burns disappeared in a couple of hours, one of hundreds of Reiki stories too numerous to fill the pages of her book. Highly recommended reading.

Susan C. Imbert, NCC, MFCC
March, 1996

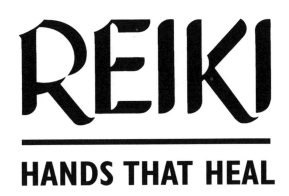

REIKI

HANDS THAT HEAL

REIKI

HANDS THAT HEAL

Joyce J. Morris, M.S., C.A.D.C.
Reiki Master Teacher

With contributor
William R. Morris, O.M.D. Reiki Master Teacher

⑨ WEISER BOOKS
York Beach, Maine, USA

First Published in 1999 by
Weiser Books
P. O. Box 612
York Beach, ME 03910-0612
www.redwheelweiser.com

Library of Congress Cataloging-in-Publication Data

Morris, Joyce J.
    Reiki hands that heal / Joyce J. Morris, with contributor William R. Morris.
      p. cm.
    Includes bibliographical references and index.
    ISBN 1-57863-118-1 (pa. : alk. paper)
    1. Reiki (Healing system)—Handbooks, manuals, etc.. 2. Mental healing—Handbooks, manuals, etc. I. Morris, William R., O.M.D. II. Title.
RZ403.R45M67 1998
615.8'52—dc21
                                             98-45654
                                             CIP

MG

Typeset in 10 pt. Palatino
Line Drawings for Reiki hand positions by Holly Bond
Printed in the United States of America

08   07   06   05   04   03   02   01
10   9   8   7   6   5   4   3

The paper used in this publication meets the minimum requirements of the American National Standard for Information Sciences—Permanence of Paper for Printed Library Materials Z39.48-1992(R1997).

Dedication

I wish to thank my parents, Gladys and Jim Jackson, for the loving supportive manner in which they raised me. Without that background of encouragement to be the best I could be, to help others, and to always stand tall, I would not be who I am today, and this book would never have been written.

To my sons, Will and Michael, from whom I have learned as much as I have taught—THANKS. A mother could not ask for finer, more loving children.

My thanks to Penelope-NiCole for her unsurpassed knowledge that she shared so freely; to Sylvia and Leonard Scruggs, for their ongoing support in all my endeavors; to my daughter-in-law, Bobbie Morris, for her constant encouragement, and to all my many students, from whom I have learned so much.

I am deeply indebted to all those who preceded me in the lineage of Reiki. To the elders of the Mystery School who used Reiki and wrote about it in the sutras; to Dr. Usui for rediscovering, and recognizing, this wonderful system; to Dr. Hayashi for having the foresight to give this knowledge to a woman, a "foreigner" who would be out of Japan when it went to war; to Madam Takata for holding this sacred knowledge safe for so many years, and then for having the wisdom to give it to Virginia Samdahl and others of her caliber so that we might have it today in its pure and ancient form.

To Virginia Samdahl, my Master, for bringing me into Reiki, for nurturing me in my growth process, for sharing her wealth of knowledge with me — I shall always be grateful.

To all my teachers, past and present, who by sharing their knowledge with me helped me to grow.

> There is one virtue above all others:
> the constant striving upwards,
> the struggle with oneself,
> the insatiable demand for greater purity,
> wisdom, goodness and love.
>
> Goethe

Table of Contents

Page

Note from the Author ix

What I Believe 1

What is Reiki 3

Reiki - The Word 7

The Reiki Story 9

The Story Continues 15

Virginia's Affirmation 17

Masters' Photos 19

Reiki Masters Lineage 29

Reiki Principles 31

Exchange of Energy 37

Professional Ethics 39

The Reiki Center 41

The Three Degrees 43

Treatment Guidelines 47

Team Treatments 51

Legal Considerations 51

The Temptations 53

Transformation Tools 55

Reiki Miracles 65

Reiki Research 71

(continued on next page)

Page

Healing Environments 77

Hand Positions 83

General Treatment Principles 121

Specific Treatments 123

Appendix A - Thesis 139

Appendix B - Research Paper 145

Appendix C - Aura Sketches 149

Appendix D - Biblical References 161

Appendix E - Addresses 163

Bibliography 165

Seminar Information 168

Index 171

About the Author 175

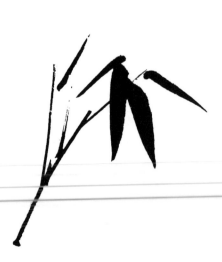

Note from the Author

This book is not meant to replace professional medical care. Be sure to secure the advice of your physician or other health care professional for any physical or emotional challenges you might have. Reiki complements many modalities of treatment; it is not meant to be used as a substitute.

This book is a self-help book in many ways. Much that you will find here will be useful to anyone on a path of spiritual growth and healing. However, reading it will NOT give you the ability to flow the Reiki energy. You cannot get Reiki by reading books, watching demonstrations or listening to a lecture. To use the Reiki energy you MUST first have Reiki attunements by a qualified Reiki Master Teacher.

What I Believe

Reiki is not a belief system.

Anyone who gets the full Reiki initiations can use the Reiki energy for healing themselves and others. Belief in Reiki is not a requirement for Reiki to work. If you get the Reiki attunements, you have the ability to flow the Reiki energy; a class, and this book—or any book—are only the packages a Master wraps Reiki in to present it to you. This book reflects MY Beliefs, my package. It stays as close as possible to the teachings I received when Reiki was passed down to me and only broadens that knowledge with new information that I have gained since becoming a Master. What I write about Reiki has not changed from what I was taught. What I write about a context for Reiki evolves as I evolve.

I believe the Principles of Healing are always the same. The Principles are not dependent upon anyone's beliefs. Since Reiki is not dependent upon a belief system, it certainly is not dependent upon your believing what I believe.

Let me start by saying that I believe in God. For me, God is NOT a man sitting on a cloud in a white robe and long white beard. That concept of God places limits based on our human ability to imagine. God is beyond limit. Nor do I believe in God as male, but as both male and female energy, so I also like to use the terms "Mother-Father God," "Divine Love," "Higher Power," "Goddess Energy," and "Spirit." To me they are just different aspects of the same loving being I call GOD.

I believe in reincarnation. I believe that we have always been, and that we will always be. I believe that this lifetime is just "a weekend vacation on earth" when placed in the context of eternity, from the beginning of time to the end of time. This is what reincarnation is all about—coming back again and again to either learn lessons, help someone, or work out Karma.

Karma, the law of cause and effect, goes along with my belief in reincarnation. I believe that some of our Karma returns to us instantly; some returns years or even lifetimes later. It can be "good" or "bad" if you give it value judgments; in truth it is simply what is. When I deal with others, if I give out love and joy and happiness, then that is what I will get in return. If, on the other hand, I give out hatred, anger and resentment, then that is what I get back. That's Karma.

Free will, on the other hand, indicates how God does NOT control us, but rather with love allows us to grow and make our own choices, make our own mistakes, and to learn from them—or not. That's up to us. As we go along in life, we are constantly at new crossroads where we must make a choice: do we go right or left? A little further down the path there will be another fork and we must choose again. Life is one choice after another, from birth until death. God does not interfere with these choices. That's free will. That is how we as individuals determine our own Karma.

I hope you find this book enjoyable, and that it broadens your knowledge of Reiki. It is important to remember, however, that only through attunements by a true Reiki Master can you be opened to flow the specific frequency of energy that is Reiki. This manual is meant primarily for my students; you may also find it interesting if you simply wish to know more about Reiki or if you are a Reiki Master and want a thorough manual for use in class. It is my hope that this book will help correct much of the misinformation that people currently have regarding Reiki, its history, what it is and what it is not. In addition, it reflects my "package"—how I see Reiki fitting into a life of healing, harmony, balance and love. In Love and Light,

1

What is Reiki?

On first encountering the word, "Reiki," most people want to know what it is and what it does. My answer can be as simple as "It's a healing energy," but since I feel strongly that the best way to find out about Reiki is to have a personal experience of the energy, I generally invite the person to a free Reiki Workshop. In a workshop, a person learns what Reiki is and what it will do—and, most important, experiences the actual energy. There are several fine books that will broaden your knowledge of Reiki,[1] but five minutes of treatment will tell more than five hours of lectures or reading.

Reiki is East meets West. It is all religions, it encompasses all religions, it is the ultimate ecumenical link. Dr. Usui, who rediscovered Reiki, was a Christian monk, studying with Zen Buddhists, going to India and the United States for additional study, then back to the Zen Master where one of his first miracles took place.[2] Reiki is based on a Master/Teacher relationship and on student initiations as the basis of learning. Western culture is growing more aware of multiple approaches to spirituality, and Reiki is a perfect melding of East and West.

Reiki is Universal Life Energy—a balanced energy flowing through the therapist that brings about healing. (It makes no difference whether we call ourselves therapists, practitioners, channels or healers. It is all the same: we flow the Reiki energy.) When I learned Reiki we were taught that it worked on 4 levels: physical, mental, emotional and spiritual. Over the years we have found evidence that it works on karmic and etheric levels, and we are getting validation that it also works on both time and space. Before we are finished learning all that Reiki is, I believe we will find that it works on 12 levels. I have no idea what the additional levels may be; it should be an interesting journey for all of us to discover these new levels.

> You are given the gifts of the gods, you create your reality according to your beliefs.
>
> Yours is the creative energy that makes your world.
>
> There are no limitations to the self except those you believe in.
>
> Jane Roberts
> —The Nature of Personal Reality

How does Reiki work on these different levels? On the physical level, Reiki helps to bring balance. When the body is in a state of balance it tends to heal itself: burns heal faster, breaks mend sooner than expected, bleeding stops, etc. On the mental level, when one is in a state of balance stress is easier to handle, learning comes easier, clarity becomes a part of everyday life, etc. With emotional balance, one is less likely to need psychiatric medication; the everyday ups and downs of life become more manageable. Spiritual growth is extremely important to many of us today, and when one is in a state of balance it is easier to meditate and pray, to listen to the inner voice and to act on higher guidance.

Karma with another individual can impede growth, and Reiki often assists the practitioner to see the karmic ties to another individual, and ways to cut or balance out the situation. Many people feel that dis-ease often begins first in the etheric web and then manifests in the physical. Reiki helps to heal rips and tears in this web and also strengthens the overall etheric web. Time and space, as well as the other 4 levels (whatever they turn out to be), are areas we are just beginning to experience.

Reiki is not learned with the conscious mind. We have memory at cellular level, and we learn all over our bodies, with every fiber of our being. The ability to flow the Reiki energy is acquired through a process done by a Reiki Master. This process is called an alignment, an attunement, or an initiation. We really do not have the vocabulary to properly describe much of what Reiki is, what it does, or how it is acquired. Since Reiki is not acquired with the conscious mind, anyone, regardless of age or mental abilities, can be attuned to the Reiki energy. The important thing to remember is that to do Reiki one must first be initiated by a Reiki Master. This is the ONLY way. It cannot be "channeled," given by one's "guides," acquired by reading or by knowledge shared by anyone other than a Master.

To become a Reiki Master one has been through the process of being initiated into First Degree, then into Second Degree, and after much time and practice has been chosen to be a Master. First and Second Degree are levels one chooses for oneself and are available to everyone. Rarely is one chosen to be a Master, for Mastership is not for everyone. At this level it is not a personal decision. If and when it is time for you to become a Master, your master will know and will tell you so, just as it has been for centuries in the Oriental martial arts and in spiritual practices.

> *Before enlightenment chopping wood carrying water.*
>
> *After enlightment carrying water chopping wood.*
>
> —Zen Proverb

Reiki has its own innate intelligence. It knows where it is needed and it goes there. Every area of the body knows its own perfection, i.e., the liver regenerates as liver cells, not as skin cells, and skin cells as skin cells not as liver cells. What Reiki does on the physical plane is to help the body return to its own perfection, whatever that might be.

What I have found is that Reiki is a harmonizing energy: it enters and balances out any imbalances within the system. When we are in a state of balance, we are healthy—both physically and emotionally. When we are out of balance, we are in a state of dis-ease. By bringing balance and harmony to the system, Reiki helps the body and the mind to heal themselves.

Reiki is a healing, balancing energy that comes through the Reiki Channel. It is NOT the practitioner's own energy, but rather a cosmic energy that enters through the crown chakra at the top of the head, flows down through the body, expands the auric field and flows out through the hands. It is drawn through in direct proportion to the amount of energy needed by the recipient, not what the therapist thinks is needed.

This has been validated for me many times over the years by many different clairvoyants, who can actually see auric fields. What they uniformly see is a funnel of white light coming in through the crown chakra; then they see the auric field expand; next they see it coming out of minor chakras in the palms of the hands and from the fingertips.

Another way I have of explaining Reiki is by comparing it to a radio. We are surrounded by radio waves at all times. If I reach out and wave my arm it goes right through radio waves. At the same time it also goes through Reiki waves. I cannot just cup my hand behind my ear and hear the radio; neither can I just reach out and tap into Reiki waves. I must have a radio, an instrument designed specifically to pick up and amplify the radio waves, in order to hear the radio. In like manner I must go through a Reiki initiation in order to pick up and amplify the Reiki energy. Reiki, like radio waves, is a vibratory energy. In the chapter on Creating an Environment we will talk much more about vibratory energies.

REIKI:

"Heals the cause and eliminates the effect," according to Madam Takata
Can be used on plants, animals, infants & children, other people, and yourself
Lasts a lifetime
Is compatible with both allopathic and homeopathic medicine
Protects the therapist from "taking on" the dis-ease of the client
Gives a treatment to the therapist as they are treating a client

Can usually be felt by both the therapist and the client, and manifests as HEAT, COLD, TINGLING, THROBBING, and a variety of other sensations.

Always works—it may not work on the area you wish, but it always works

Always works, but the client may not stay with it long enough to effect a "cure" or change in the problem

Makes a statement to the Universe that you are WORTH healing, and that rather than going to someone else and saying, "Here I am, fix me," you are taking RESPONSIBILITY for your own health and well-being

REIKI IS:

A GREAT stress reducer
Simple and easy to use
A "psychic roto-rooter"
Compatible with all religions
Easy to learn, easier to use
A release for blocked energy
Safe

REIKI IS NOT:

A religion
A belief system
Hypnosis or mind control
Psychic Healing
Laying-on-of-hands
Learned with the conscious mind

ACCORDING TO WILLIAM MORRIS, O.M.D.:

Reiki is pure undifferentiated life force; as such, it is pure goodness.

Reiki is that life force which exists before polarization into yin and yang and the 10,000 things; as such, it is close to the Tao.

As a nonpolarized energy, Reiki is attracted to where polarized imbalances exist.

As universal life force in expression, Reiki is a quantum form of healing.

Reiki is a form of healing which emanates from the absolute.

Reiki is an unconditional form of healing.

Reiki reveals the innate gift of healing which is the human birth-right. As such, it is a consummate expression of love.

Reiki reveals the body's innate intelligence to heal itself.

The gift of Reiki is a gift of supreme satisfaction.

---

1. See bibliography.
2. The history of Reiki is covered in "The Story Continues," p. 15.

We are not here just to survive
and live long...

We are here to live and know life
in its multi-dimensions
to know life in its richness,
in all its variety.

And when a man lives multi-
dimensionally, explores all
possibilities available,
never shrinks back
from any challenge,

Goes, rushes to it, welcomes it,
rises to the occasion
then life becomes a flame,
life blooms.

Bhagwan Shree Rajneesh

6

Reiki - The Word

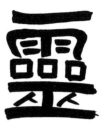
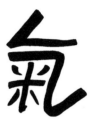

Reiki is pronounced—

Ray as a Ray of Light

Key as a Key to unlock a door

The dictionary gives varied meanings of the word. Some of them are:

Rei - Spirit, Soul, Universal

Ki - Energy

Together they could mean "Soul Energy" or "Spirit Energy." However, the essence is more that of Universal Life Energy.

Ki has a name in most languages:

- In Chinese, Chi or Qi
- Christ Light to Christians
- Prana in Hindu
- Bioplasma in Russia
- Mana to Hawaiian Kahunas
- Orgone Energy to Wilhelm Reich
- In English, the Breath of Life, Vital Life Force Energy, Ectoplasm, Bio-Energetics.

On the certificate you receive at the completion of class, you will see, "USUI SHIKI RYOHO." This translates into "The Usui System of Natural Healing."

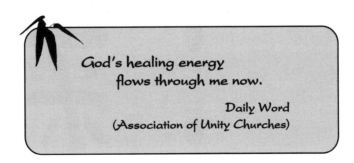

God's healing energy
flows through me now.

Daily Word
(Association of Unity Churches)

To help increase our understanding of Reiki, where it comes from and what it means, we have an explanation of the Reiki symbol by William Morris, O.M.D.

This entire character (both Rei and Ki together) is used in very ancient medical texts. It has been found in manuscripts dating from two and three thousand B.C.

About that time in most cultures the two classes, priests and physicians, became divided. Before then the spiritual leaders were also the healers.

In the Orient, the physicians took the Reiki character out and inserted another character which symbolizes herbs or potions or some physical substance that they would give to the people.

The first portion of the symbol is Rei

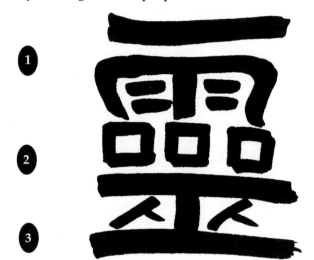

1. The upper section of the character is a cloud formation or condensation of energy. It represents an all-prevailing energy and what it shows is a coming together and focusing of the energy.

2. The middle section is under the cloud formations. These are 3 squares which represent people with open hungry mouths.

3. Below the squares are stick figures that symbolize priests performing ceremony.

This part of the story tells of the people beseeching the priests to bring rain.

The second part of the symbol is Ki, and this is a very specific form of Ki. In some ancient medical texts there are as many as 38 different forms of Ki or Chi manifestations. These range from breathing vital life force to basic organ functions. This character represents grains or other nutrients coming out of the earth.

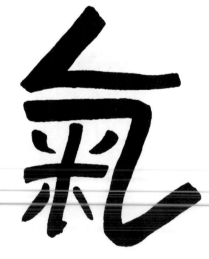

1. The whole symbol is a vortex of energy.

2. The cross is symbolic of a patch of earth or ground.

3. These four little sprouts are rice.

This is the essence of Reiki—a balance of heaven, earth and humanity—a concept which is intrinsic to Chinese thought.

The Reiki Story

In the mid-1800s, **Dr. Mikao Usui** was head of a Christian School, comparable to a theological seminary in the U.S., in Kyoto, Japan. His students were constantly asking him why they were only being taught to heal the soul when the Bible says it is possible to heal both the body and the soul. Dr. Usui did not have an answer for them, and he felt he was compelled to.

He left his position at the school and went on a lengthy search, which took him to several countries, including the United States. He learned several languages in the progress of his travels so he could study each culture's manuscripts in their original form instead of in translations.

After long years of searching, Dr. Usui finally found what he was sure were the keys for physical healing and balancing in the Sanskrit sutras (the word "sutras" simply means "holy writings"). What he found was a formula, very clear and precise, for a simple, quick, easy way to activate and direct the Universal Life Energy that he later named Reiki. What he did not find was the way to get the power to start the activation. He conferred with the abbot of the Zen Buddhist monastery where he was staying; they decided he should go up onto Mount Kurama-yama, a sacred mountain outside Kyoto, for 21 days of meditation, prayer, and fasting to see if he could gain the power he sought.

> Ask, and it shall be given you,
> seek, and ye shall find,
> knock, and it shall be opened
> unto you:
> For every one that asketh
> receiveth,
> and he that seeketh
> findeth,
> and to him that knocketh
> it shall be opened.
>
> Matthew 7:7-8
> —King James Bible

To keep track of the days, Dr. Usui gathered up 21 stones. Each day he threw away one of the stones, and then he meditated, prayed, read from the sutras, and fasted. Finally the morning of the 21st day came. We are told that before dawn he said:

"My Father, my God, this is the morning of the twenty-first day. I pray you will show me the light." And I threw the stone away.

And in that way over on the horizon, as he did that, he saw a little bitty beam of light. And it started moving towards him. As it moved, it came faster and faster and got larger and larger and it frightened him nearly to death.

He jumped to his feet and turned to run, as he was really afraid! He thought to himself, "If that hits me, it'll kill me!"

*Then he caught himself. And he swung around and shouted "No! I have spent years in my search. I have just asked to be shown the light. I will **not** run away!"*

He placed his feet and braced himself, and said, "Father, if it kills me, I'll accept the light." And he said that when he made that decision, this light simply burst upon him. It struck him in the middle of his forehead and knocked him to the ground, unconscious. And he told Hyashi that he believed that at that moment he died.

The next thing he knew, he saw bubbles . . . millions and millions of bubbles all moving from right to left in every color of the rainbow. From the palest pink to the deepest cerise; from the palest green to the deepest emerald; palest aqua to the deepest blue. And after all these gorgeous colors the gold came, and in the gold the white lights. And in the center of every white bubble was a gold figure in the Sanskrit that he had learned and read in the **Sutras.**

And the bubble would come and stop, as though it would say, "Here, Usui, learn this so you will know it always and be able to use it." And it would go. And then another would come and stop. And he was so afraid that he'd miss something that he told Hyashi he didn't even blink!

Finally he felt he had it all, and said, "Thank you, God. Now I have it. I know I can use it. Thank you, thank you, thank you."

And he said the next thing he knew, he opened his eyes and it was broad daylight! It was the middle of the morning.

And then he thought, "Ahhhhh! What a fantastic experience!"[1]

And so started the miracles that Dr. Usui was to experience. Filled with wonder and excitement, he dusted the pine needles, dust, and dirt off his clothes, and suddenly realized a **miracle** had occurred—he was not weak and tired, even after 21 days of fasting.

In his excitement, Dr. Usui took off running down the mountain and, in his eagerness, stubbed his toe. It was very painful and bleeding, so he sat down and held it for a while. He soon realized that the palms of his hands had become very hot and the pain and throbbing in his toe had stopped. When he looked he found that the bleeding had stopped also—the toe was totally healed. The **second Reiki miracle** had occurred.

On his way down the mountainside he realized he was extremely hungry. He came upon a bench covered with a red blanket and with an ashtray in the middle. In the mountains of Japan this means welcome, there is fast food service here. So he sat down and ordered a big breakfast.

While he was waiting for his breakfast, the little daughter of the owner came out of the house crying, her face swollen and wrapped with a large rag tied at the top of her head. She told Dr. Usui that she had had a toothache for days, but it was too far to go into Kyoto to the dentist and they were too poor to afford to go. Dr. Usui had her sit in front of him and he put a hand on each side of her face. She soon excitedly told him he had done MAGIC, his hands were hot and the pain and swelling was gone. This healing was **Reiki miracle number three.**

Soon the man came out with a big breakfast that included raw fish, pickled plums, and other delicacies, food he had tried to talk Dr. Usui out of eating. He knew that with Dr. Usui just coming off a fast the food should be bland, but Dr. Usui was not to be put off, for he was famished. He ate his lavish breakfast and suffered no indigestion: **Reiki miracle number four.**

When Dr. Usui arrived back at the monastery he was told the Bishop was in bed with a bad attack of arthritis. As soon as he had cleaned up and gotten some food he went to tell the Bishop of his adventures. While talking to the Bishop he put one of his hands on the Bishop's back and one on his hip. Soon the pain was gone and the **fifth Reiki miracle** had taken place.

That night Dr. Usui and the Bishop prayed and meditated so they could determine what should be done with the Reiki. Over breakfast the next morning it was decided that Dr. Usui should go to Beggar City and heal the beggars. Once they were healed, Dr. Usui believed that they could go to the temple, get new names (as was the custom when beginning a new life), and start new lives for themselves.

Dr. Usui dressed as a beggar so he would fit in better and be more readily accepted, and down to Beggar City he went. For seven years he worked with the beggars. He treated them, he healed them, and many more miracles occurred.

One night he was out walking around and he saw a familiar face. When he asked the young man why he looked familiar—

> The young man said, "Ah, Dr. Usui. You know me. Of course you know me. I'm one of the first fellows that you healed down here!"
>
> Usui exclaimed, "I healed you? **I healed you?** If I healed you, what are you doing here? I sent you out to make a new name, to make a new life!"
>
> And he said, "Oh I did that."
>
> "You did that?"
>
> He said, "Sure. But do you know how much self-discipline it takes to get up and go to work every day? Do you know how hard I had to work for just a few pennies? And we were **still** hungry all the time. I would rather be a beggar!"
>
> And Usui sank to his knees. "What, oh what have I done? The churches were right. A person has to be healed of spirit as well as of body. Reiki given away makes beggars of people!"
>
> And he dropped to the ground and just rubbed his head into the dirt.
>
> Then he stood up and said, "I cut off all beggars. Never again will Reiki be given away. Always the flow will have to be completed. Always there will have to be an exchange with Reiki. And now I know how to heal the body **and** the spirit—"
>
> And he knocked the dirt of Beggar City off his feet, and went back up to Kyoto.[2]

Looking back over his seven years in Beggar City he realized he had forgotten to teach them the spiritual side of healing. He had forgotten to teach them gratitude. At this time Dr. Usui formulated the Five Principles of Reiki.

When Dr. Usui got back to Kyoto, he found a very large torch, and, early the next morning, he went to the busiest corner in all of Kyoto, lit his torch, and started walking around. People stared and laughed at him for holding a lit torch in broad daylight. Finally a young man asked Dr. Usui why he was holding a torch on such a bright, sunny day.

> And Usui said, "You see that torch? That is because I am hunting for people who do not want illness in a home, who do not want to have a lot of big doctors' bills, who want to learn how to live in a good fun-fulfilled life. And if you want to know the story of Reiki, you come to that temple over there at 7 o'clock tonight and you can bring all of that into your life.[3]

And so began Dr. Usui's travels. From this time on, until his transition in the early 1900's, he traveled throughout Japan lecturing and teaching Reiki. On his travels he acquired 18 disciples, young men who traveled and studied with him. And so began a tradition of apprenticeship in Reiki.

Dr. Usui had two children, but they did not want to dedicate their lives to Reiki, so when it was time for him to make his transition he chose **Dr. Chujiro Hayashi,** his most dedicated disciple, to carry on the tradition of Reiki.

Dr. Hayashi was a member of the Japanese aristocracy, a very learned and enlightened man, and an Admiral in the Japanese Naval Reserve. After Dr. Usui's transition, he started a Reiki clinic in Tokyo which flourished for many years. Like Dr. Usui, Dr. Hayashi also had two children (a boy and a girl) who were not interested in dedicating their lives to Reiki.

Before his transition, he chose **Hawayo Takata** to be the next person to hold in trust the sacred knowledge of Reiki. What safer place to hide this precious knowledge when his country was about to go to war, than with a woman, who would not be called upon to bear arms, and who lived in Hawaii instead of Japan, and therefore was an American citizen.

The year was 1941; as a clairvoyant Dr. Hayashi saw what was about to happen to his country. Not wanting to go to war (for he was now a healer, not a warrior), he gathered all of his family, students and friends together, and had a farewell gathering. When he had finished with his farewells he closed his eyes, whispered, "There, I have broken my aorta," and left his body. The date was May 10, 1941. Many people aspire to reach this level of enlightenment—the ability to leave the body at will, rather than having to have an accident or a dis-ease. Although many aspire to this level, very few reach it. Dr. Hayashi did.

Hawayo K. Takata was born on December 24, 1900, the second daughter of Japanese sugar cane workers. Her mother named her Hawayo in honor of the big island of Hawaii. Takata grew up working first in the cane fields and later in the main plantation house. Her formal education ended at the second grade. Takata was trained to work in the main house where she met the family accountant, Saichi Takata. Hawayo and Saichi fell in love and were soon married. With a loving husband and two growing daughters her life seemed wonderful, until at age 31 she was widowed. The burden was too great for her and soon her health began to falter. In the mid-1930s she took her daughters to Japan so her parents could care for them when she died. After a few months of rest at her parents home, she was in good enough health to undergo surgery.

As she lay on the operating table waiting for the surgery, she heard a voice tell her the operation was not necessary. She thought she was going crazy—hearing voices when no one was around. When, for the third time, she heard the voice say the operation was not necessary, she asked it what she should do, and she was told to "ask the Doctor." Takata confronted her doctor, told him she didn't think the surgery was necessary, and asked him if he knew of any other kind of treatment for her condition. Recently the doctor's sister had been healed by another doctor in Tokyo, one who used drugless and bloodless treatments, so he referred Takata there.

Takata was taken to the Reiki Clinic run by Dr. Chujiro Hayashi. There were eight beds and sixteen therapists. Each day Takata received a full Reiki treatment and her health slowly returned. Within 8 months she was totally healed and her life was transformed. She wanted to be able to help others with this wonderful healing energy, but Dr. Hayashi told her no, healing was a man's domain, prohibited to women, particularly women of the working class.

Takata persisted and Dr. Hayashi resisted. She stayed and helped out at the clinic, doing errands and whatever chores needed to be done. Finally, in the spring of 1936, Dr. Hayashi relented and initiated Takata as the first woman, the first non-Japanese, and the first relatively uneducated person to have First Degree Reiki. Takata took her daughters and returned to Hawaii where she spent her time healing herself, her family, and friends.

On a trip to Hawaii with his daughter, when Dr. Hayashi found out all Takata had been doing with her Reiki, he broke with tradition again and initiated Takata into Second Degree Reiki. In the winter of 1938, before returning to Japan, Dr. Hayashi paid Takata the ultimate honor of bestowing upon her the knowledge of Reiki Mastership—the last person to be initiated by Dr. Hayashi himself. In order to reach this level Takata had to sell her home, the only thing she had of value, to raise the $10,000 that Dr. Hayashi had set for Reiki Mastership, based upon the amount he had paid for his Mastership. That exchange is honored to this day by true Reiki Masters.

For many years Takata devoted herself to teaching Reiki and to treating anyone who was ill. For years she traveled throughout the islands, and in the 1950s made a few trips to the United States. She came as a personal friend and companion to Doris Duke, the tobacco heiress. During this time she trained Mrs. Duke and a few of her friends, including Aldous Huxley.[4] Students at that time were told never to tell anyone that they had Reiki. This was sacred knowledge that Takata felt must be kept secret; she felt the time was not yet right for the world to know about Reiki.

In the early 1970s Takata started teaching extensively in the United States. In 1974 she trained **Virginia Samdahl** at First Degree, in 1975 at Second Degree, and in 1976 as the first Occidental Reiki Master. Before her transition in December of 1980, at the age of 80, Takata trained a total of 22 Master Teachers. Takata's grandaughter, Phyllis Lei Furumoto, is the current head of the Reiki lineage.

READING LIST
Students may want to read the following titles in relation to this chapter: Arnold & Nevius, *The Reiki Handbook*; Brown, *Living Reiki*; Haberly, *Reiki: Hawayo Takata's Story*; Baginsky & Sharonon, *Reiki: Universal Life Energy*; Eos, *Reiki and Medicine*; Stuart, *The Reiki Touch*. See Bibliography for publisher information.

---

1. Larry E. Arnold and Sandra K. Nevius, *The Reiki Handbook* (Harrisburg, PA: PSI Press, 1992), 4th edition, p. 7.
2. Larry E. Arnold and Sandra K. Nevius, *The Reiki Handbook*, pp. 10-11.
3. Larry E. Arnold and Sandra K. Nevius, *The Reiki Handbook*, p. 11.
4. Personal communication with Phyllis and Sidney Krystal, 1985, in Los Angeles. Both had been students of Takata's in the 1950s in Los Angeles: Phyllis at 2nd Degree, Sidney at 1st Degree.

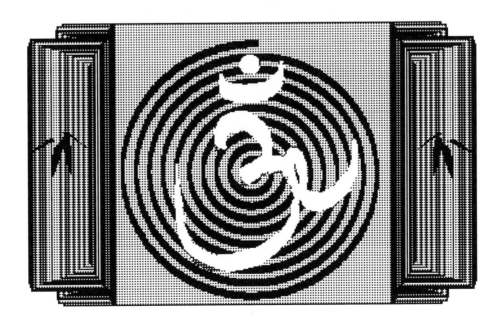

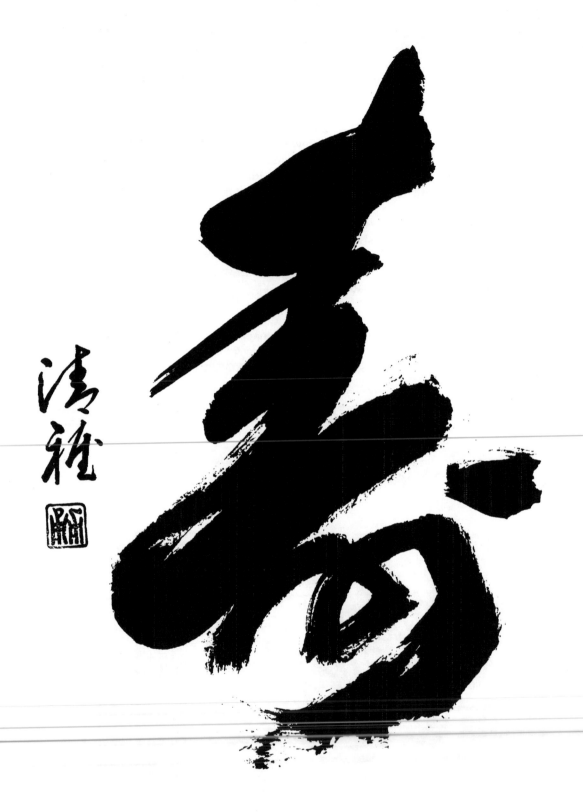

(Long Life)

The Story Continues...

Virginia Samdahl[1] had been a healer and a teacher of metaphysics for many years before she was introduced to Reiki. When she was introduced to Reiki, she realized she had finally found what she was looking for—a healing modality that always works, one that can ease the process of transition, quiet the pain in dis-eases that usually cause great pain, bring "remission" in some instances, full healing in others, and enhance spiritual growth and transformation.

Virginia's experiences with parapsychology began when she was a young child. After the tragic death of her younger son, Walker, Virginia joined a healing prayer group and started to develop her natural talents of clairaudience, clairvoyance, and precognition. Before long this developed into the ability to do spirit communication and healing. Although her husband, Leo, was not personally interested in parapsychological activities, he was very supportive of Virginia's work. They had two children in addition to Walker, another son Lee, and a daughter Adair.

After becoming a Reiki Master, Virginia traveled extensively teaching Reiki. She was very active in the Spiritual Frontiers Fellowship, and taught at their functions for many years before retiring.

In February of 1981, two months after Madam Takata's transition, I was introduced to Reiki. I was working at the time as an alcoholism and drug counselor in Springfield, Ohio, and was constantly searching for better stress management tools to use with my clients. I had read several books on foot reflexology and felt I could easily teach this to my clients, so, when I heard of someone who did reflexology treatments, I called for an appointment. When I got there the man said he and his wife had just studied Reiki, and could they give me a Reiki treatment? Willing to try almost anything I said sure, as long as I could still get my reflexology treatment, since I needed that experience to be able to teach my clients to do reflexology on themselves. Well—within 5 minutes I said, "I don't know what you're doing, but I must have it, I've never felt so relaxed, so fast, in all my life."

As soon as Virginia came to town I took my First Degree. I had absolutely no intention of going any further in Reiki. I had recently paid off all the debts left me in a divorce, and on my salary could not imagine paying $500 for Second Degree. By the time Virginia came back to town I was more than ready to pay whatever it would cost to get the added knowledge Second Degree offered. I had parents living in south Georgia, both my sons living in California, and both my private and agency practice as an alcoholism and drug counselor had grown by leaps and bounds, and I NEEDED what Second Degree could bring.

> Be realistic:
> Plan for a miracle.
>
> Bhagwan Shree Rajneesh

The following year when Virginia told me I was to be a Master I told her that the idea was crazy. I had no idea if Reiki was to be my spiritual path. I was content with my life. I did not want to make the changes necessary if I were to become a Master (also there was no way I could pay $10,000, or even close to it). She kept insisting that I should interview with the Board of the A.R.A (American Reiki Association), and also talk with Phyllis Furumoto, head of the Reiki Alliance, the only initiators of Masters at that time. After both interviews, it became obvious what the Universe wanted, for I was chosen and the money manifested in strange and wondrous ways. I chose to train with Barbara Ray and the A.R.A.[2] because I felt I needed their more structured program.

In the fall I completed my Masters training and had the thrill of giving my first Reiki attunements to my parents and my sons. Both sons had been on spiritual paths for some time and were also accomplished astrologers and metaphysicians. Neither was expecting anything special from this "thing" that Mom had learned back in Ohio. Were they surprised! Soon all their friends wanted Reiki and so my teaching on the West Coast began. By the next spring we opened the first Reiki Center in Los Angeles.

---

1. Barbara D. Lugenbeel, *Virginia Samdahl: Reiki Master Healer* (Norfolk, VA: Grunwald and Radcliff, 1984).
2. The A.R.A. later became the A.I.R.A. (American International Reiki Association) and is sometimes known as the Radiance Technique.

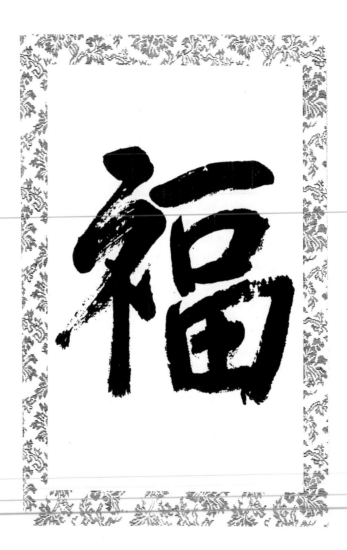

Reiki is God's Love in its purest form.

It is completely unconditional.

It demands nothing of the giver
nor of the receiver.

It propounds no creed or dogma.

It requires no specific belief in
the supreme being or in
reiki itself.
Used in its traditional form, as
developed by Dr. Usui in
the Usui System of Natural Healing,
reiki heals the body and emotions,
bringing them into balance
and promoting health, happiness,
prosperity,
and
long life.

Virginia Samdahl

Virginia's Affirmation

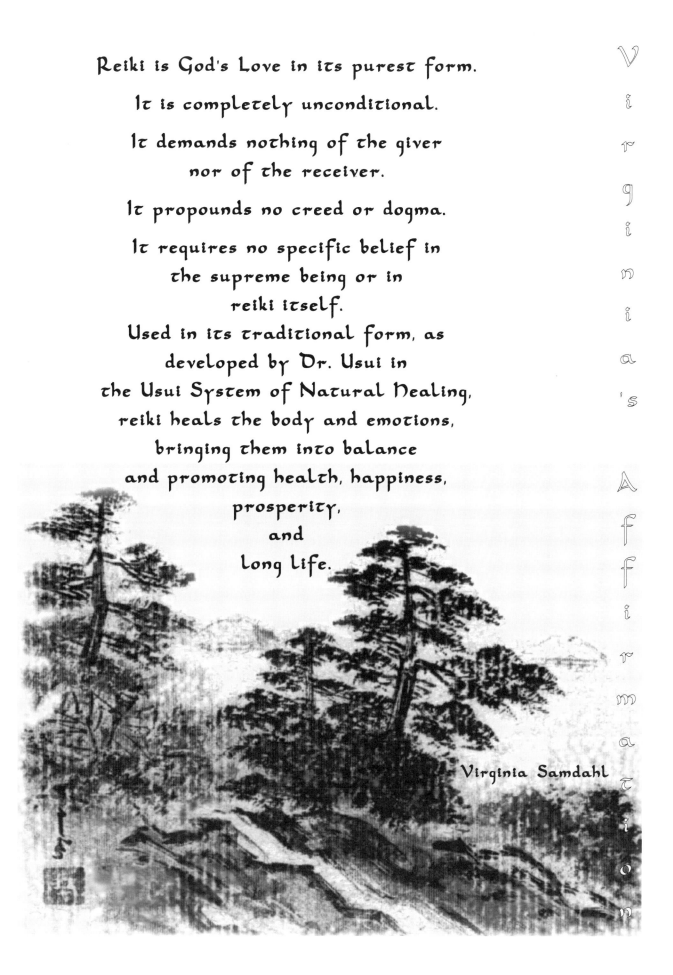

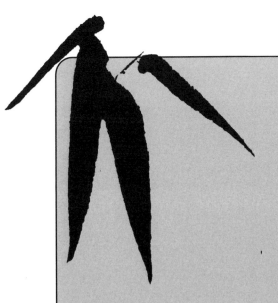

Masters' Photos

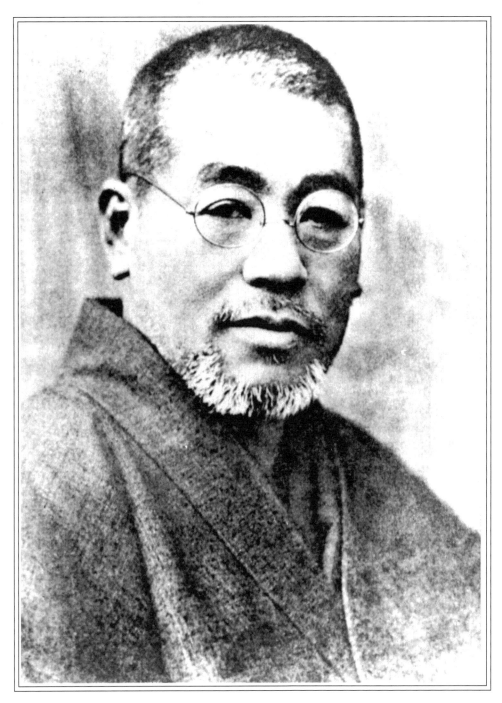

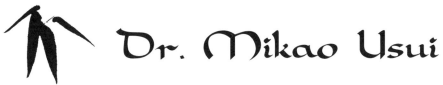

Dr. Mikao Usui

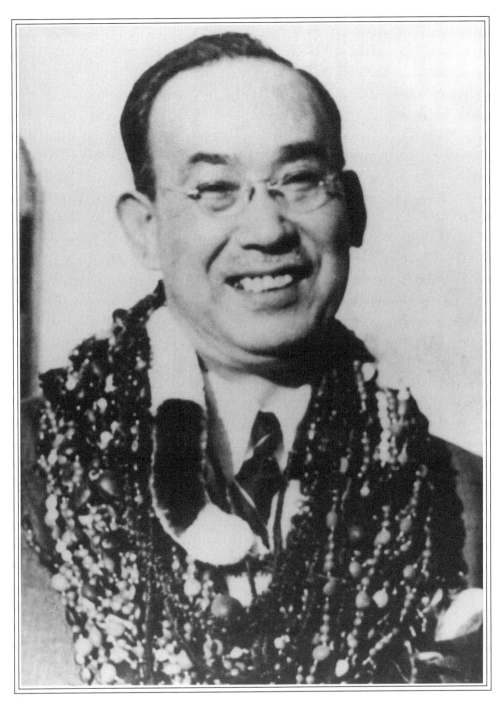

Dr. Chujiro Hayashi

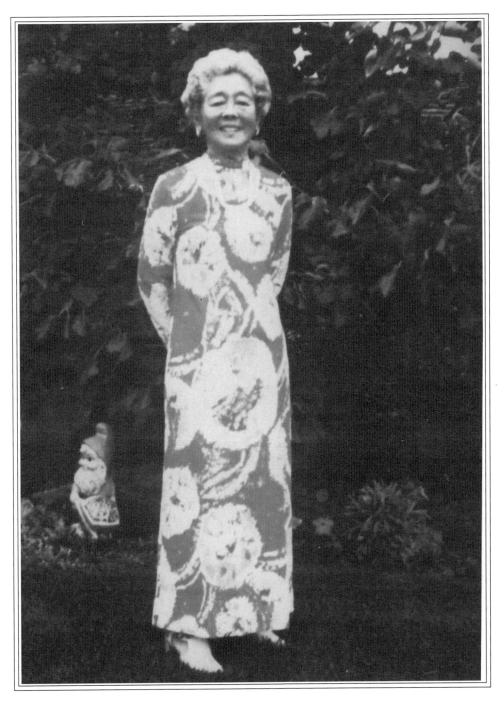

Hawayo Takata

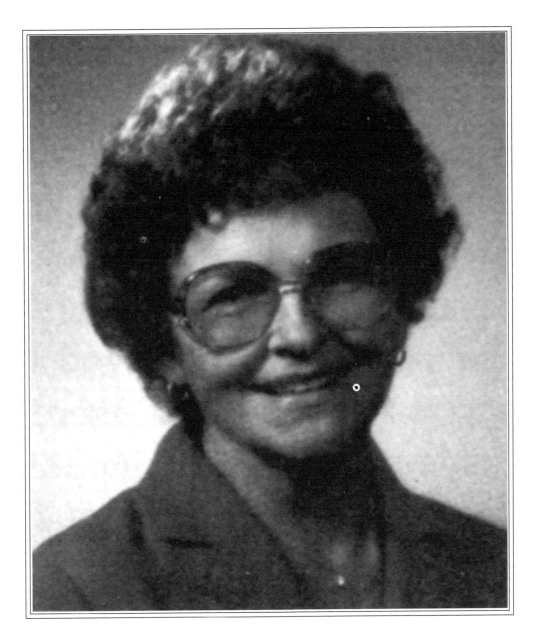

Virginia Samdahl

Reiki Masters Lineage

Dr. Mikao Usui was the person who rediscovered Reiki in the mid-1800s. Before he made his transition, he trained and initiated Dr. Chujiro Hayashi.

Dr. Hayashi trained and initiated Madam Takata. In the last ten years of her life, Madam Takata, in her turn, initiated 22 Masters before her transition in 1980. These Masters are:

> George Araki
> Dorothy Baba (transcended)
> Ursula Baylow
> Rick Bockner
> Barbara Brown
> Fran Brown
> Patricia Ewing
> Phyllis Lei Furumoto
> Beth Gray
> John Gray
> Iris Ishikura (transcended)
> Harry Kuboi
> Ethel Lombardi
> Barbara McCullough
> Mary McFadyen
> Paul Mitchell
> Bethel Phaigh (transcended)
> Barbara Weber Ray
> Shinobu Saito
> Virginia Samdahl (transcended)
> Wanja Twan
> Sister of Mme. Takata (transcended)

You may hear many rumors of other masters trained by Madam Takata. I have heard stories of Masters coming from Africa to bring Reiki to Third World countries; of two monks/Reiki Masters in Europe coming forth after 40 years of silence to teach; of monks trained by Dr. Usui who are sitting on the side of mountains in Tibet or Nepal—and the stories go on and on. Although these stories seem plausible, when you attempt to trace the sources of these rumors, you usually find a dead end, no link to the lineage of the original 22 Masters. Only through direct connection to these 22 Masters is there true Reiki.

Unfortunately, in Reiki today you must rely on the old adage, "Let the buyer beware." The word "Reiki" is becoming almost a generic term for any type of energy work, or initiation. Anyone can claim to be a Reiki Master or to be connected to the lineage. This does not make it so. (As an example, I am aware of several people who claim I initiated them as Masters, when in fact I have either never heard of them, or I did train them, but at lower levels, NOT as Master Teachers.)

The two national organizations, The Reiki Alliance and The American International Reiki Association, only govern their own members. To be sure you are dealing with a legitimate Master, check with these organizations to be sure the person you wish to study with is a member of one of them. This is the best insurance that you are getting pure Reiki and not some mixture or the creation of someone's imagination. Another indication is that true Masters will never, ever provide what is essentially "Mastership for sale," making "Masters" of anyone who asks and pays their (usually discounted) fee. Reiki is such a phenomenal energy that it is worth carefully searching out the lineage of the person you are considering as your Master. Only pure Reiki will give you the phenomenal results we all hold so dear.

Reiki Initiations are Sacred Ceremonies that pass the spiraling healing power of Reiki from the Master to the student. These Sacred Ceremonies have come down through this pure lineage to Reiki Masters today, and we have been intrusted with their care and safekeeping so that never again will the planet be without this ancient sacred knowledge.

What is firmly established cannot
be uprooted.
What is firmly grasped cannot
slip away.
It will be honored from
generation to generation.

Cultivate Virtue in your self,
And Virtue will be real.
Cultivate it in the family,
And Virtue will abound.
Cultivate it in the village,
And Virtue will grow.
Cultivate it in the nation,
And Virtue will be abundant.
Cultivate it in the universe,
And Virtue will be everywhere.

Therefore look at the body as
body,
Look at the family as family,
Look at the village as village,
Look at the nation as nation,
Look at the universe as universe.

How do I know the universe is
like this?
By looking!

Lao Tsu
—Tao Te Ching

Reiki Principles

Dr. Usui left Beggar City because he realized that Reiki fit differently into the world than he had first thought.

He realized he had been treating only the physical, and had not been concerned with the Spiritual—the exact opposite of his teaching experiences at the University. He had not taught the Beggars gratitude. By giving away the Reiki, Dr. Usui had played into the mentality of the beggars' wanting something for nothing. They had not committed themselves to wanting the healing; they had not asked for it nor had they indicated its value to them by some exchange of energy.

We cannot assume that what we want for another person, no matter how well-intentioned, is what is truly right for them. For example, we might want a person to be "healed" so he or she does not experience pain or make their transition. The truth is that despite our best intentions, we do not know what that person's soul path is meant to be. It is possible that the soul's choice is to make its transition, using the illness to facilitate the process. Perhaps the pain (be it physical or emotional) is helping the person learn a lesson. In addition, he or she may be getting some type of benefit, such as attention from a loved one or financial support, because of the illness and may not be ready to let it go. With Reiki, the requirement is that a person desire a healing and pay for it in an appropriate manner.

> Letting go and letting God,
> I unite myself
> with divine power and authority.
> Daily Word
> (Association of Unity Churches)

Our lessons in life come in many forms, and, as with Dr. Usui, often our clarity only comes in hindsight. We create our own worlds with our thoughts, words, and actions. Usually we do it unknowingly, just as Dr. Usui did. Both Usui and the beggars learned much as a result of his seven years in Beggar City. On the surface, this experience would appear to some to be a failure, but we learn our lessons in numerous ways. (For example, I find that many people at this time are learning lessons of discernment. The lesson often is not visible until they have acted without discernment, and only through hindsight can they see the error of their ways. The '90s is definitely a period for this particular lesson. For the '70s it seemed to be "opening up"; for the '80s, "acceptance." I wonder what the next century will bring forth as its major lesson.)

> If we turn the spirit inward, we acquire the power of discernment. Through the power of discernment we find our way to the truth.
> Ramakrishna

As a result of Dr. Usui's experiences he developed a set of Principles which still hold true today. These Principles are wonderful tools to assist in the growth process. The original Five Principles of Reiki as formulated by Dr. Usui, and handed down to us today, are:

**Just for today I will give thanks for my many blessings
Just for today I will not worry
Just for today I will not be angry
Just for today I will do my work honestly
Just for today I will be kind to my neighbor and every living thing**

I love and honor these Principles and the oral tradition that brought them to us. However, with what we now know about the power of affirmations to create our reality, it may be wise to rephrase them into more positive statements. We might say:

Just for today I will give thanks for my many blessings
Just for today I will look at the positive
Just for today I will deal with anger appropriately
Just for today I will do my work honestly
Just for today I will be kind to everyone and everything.

"Just for today I will give thanks for my many blessings"

Learning to give thanks for everything in your life, the challenges as well as the joys, can turn your life around. Alcoholics Anonymous has a slogan, "Have an attitude of gratitude," that has assisted many in changing their negative attitudes into positive ones. Reiki is one of the blessings of this lifetime that we can truly give thanks for on a daily basis. To truly live in a state of gratitude, you must consciously look for the blessings. Reiki will assist in opening your consciousness so you can be aware of all that is around you just ready and waiting to be seen and appreciated.

"Just for today I will look at the positive"

When you look at the positive you will find that situations are not necessarily what they had appeared to be before. This is really a matter of looking at the glass half-full instead of half-empty. When you learn to take a positive attitude there will be less and less of the negative for you to see. When we are in a negative state of mind, we are indicating a lack of faith in God to take care of us. Negativity and worry don't help anything—they just hinder the outcome, and make us miserable in the meantime. Learn to do your groundwork, turn the results over to God, or a Higher Power of your understanding, and you will find yourself naturally becoming more positive.

"Just for today I will deal with anger appropriately"

To say we will not be angry is difficult, for there are some things in life that we have every right to be angry about. However, **how** we handle that anger is what is important. Anger is really an "umbrella" emotion, usually covering up feelings of hurt, frustration, or resentment. A major step forward in many people's growth path is learning to develop skills to uncover and deal with the emotions that are hidden behind this label, and take action for change if that is what is necessary. When they can deal appropriately with the anger, their lives become much happier.

"Just for today I will do my work honestly"

Doing your work honestly, whether for yourself or another, is crucial for good self esteem. You can sometimes fool other people with dishonesty, but you cannot fool yourself. You are the one who must look at yourself in the mirror each morning. Doing your work honestly, and in a larger sense living your life honestly, knowing that your ethics are clean whether anyone else knows or not, brings you peace of mind you can find no other way. The daily decisions to live ethically may be difficult but the serenity that results transforms lives.

"Just for today I will be kind to everyone and everything"

Reiki is an energy of the heart. When you are giving Reiki, you will naturally be kind, since kindness and love walk hand in hand. Again, since we create our own worlds, attempting to be kind and loving to everyone and everything around you will create a loving atmosphere for you to live in as well.

And this is what we call

Living

Reiki!

Just for today
I will give thanks
for my many blessings

Just for today
I will not worry

Just for today
I will not be angry

Just for today
I will do my work honestly

Just for today
I will be kind
to my neighbor
and every living thing.

Dr. Mikao Usui

Just for today
I will give thanks
for my many blessings

Just for today
I will look at the positive

Just for today
I will deal with anger
appropriately

Just for today
I will do my work honestly

Just for today
I will be kind to everyone
and everything.

Joyce Morris

Exchange of Energy

Whenever we are dealing with energy, it is very important to keep it flowing equally, in both directions. I'm sure you all know of relationships where one person does all the giving, and the other all the taking. This makes for a very unhealthy relationship. This kind of "control" trap can happen with Reiki, so it is important that there **always** be a fair exchange of energy. This can be money, barter, or the natural give-and-take within a close family or friendship setting. Dr. Usui found in Beggar City that those who received Reiki without giving something in exchange did not honor it, and therefore did not have a permanent healing. This is why Dr. Usui said,

> *I cut off all beggars. Never again will Reiki be given away. Always the flow will have to be completed. Always there will have to be an exchange with Reiki.*[1]

In reality, when we are willing to give, but not willing to receive, what we are actually doing is trying to control another. It is never wise to make another human being "indebted" to you, for when you do, you are creating a Karmic situation that is not just for this lifetime, but for all eternity—until it is balanced out. It is better not to create the Karma in the first place.

Many people have difficulty charging for Reiki treatments. They feel no one should charge for a healing, especially a spiritual healing. What they forget is that they are not charging for a healing. REIKI does the healing—they are just charging for their time. It might be great if everything in life were free, however at present the landlord and mortgage company want money, not cherry pie, in payment each month; the grocer wants money in exchange for the food you buy; the clothes you need to keep you both warm and presentable cost money. Remember, "time is money," and "the laborer is worthy of his hire."

> Declaring that divine order prevails in all blesses me everywhere J go and in all that J do.
>
> Jn the overall plan, divine order is perfect balance – the right relation of all people and all things one to another.
>
> Daily Word
> (Association of Unity Churches)

Much of our thinking about money is not ours, but rather ideas we have been handed down from our Puritan forefathers. Don't let beliefs in poverty, lack, and limitation hold you, or anyone else, back from their good. When your PROSPERITY CONSCIOUSNESS is where it should be, you will have no difficulty charging for treatments, and charging what they are worth. Money is just a means of exchange—it fits in the wallet or purse a lot easier than a cherry pie.[2]

Reiki is a great service, or tool, to use for barter. A Reiki treatment usually is priced at the same rate as a massage in the area where it is given. When you barter a treatment, the exchange should be equal in value. I know someone who bartered with her dentist for major dental work, another who bartered for maintenance on her car, another who has a credit at the local health food restaurant every week. You are limited only by your imagination. Have fun!

Occasionally there may be times when it is inappropriate to be paid or to barter for a Reiki treatment. In these situations, for example, when coming upon a highway accident, it is quite appropriate to give Reiki as a donation to the Universe. I use an affirmation that I would like to share with you to accomplish this. By using this, or some other affirmation, you will not be putting yourself in the position of attempting to control another human being—for we never know what the soul's choice might be.

I freely, and with Love, donate this treatment to the universe, activating the law of ten-fold return, accepting my good in whatever present form is best.

1. Larry E. Arnold and Sandra K. Nevius, *The Reiki Handbook* (Harrisburg, PA: PSI Press, 1992), 4th Edition, p. 11.
2. See "Transformation Tools," p. 55.

We draw spiritual substance to ourselves just as the magnet draws the iron. When we think about the love of God drawing to us the substance necessary for support and supply, that substance begins to accumulate all around us, and as we abide in the consciousness of it, it begins to manifest itself in all our affairs.

Fear is a great breeder of poverty, for it breaks down positive thoughts. Negative thoughts bring negative conditions in their train. The first thing to do in making a demonstration of prosperity in the home is to discard all negative thoughts and words. Build up a positive thought atmosphere in the home, an atmosphere that is free from fear and filled with love. Do not allow any words of poverty or lack to limit the attractive power of love in the home.

Unity Magazine
(Association of Unity Churches)

Professional Ethics

Never diagnose or prescribe unless you are licensed to do so (i.e., an M.D., Chiropractor, Acupuncturist, D.O., etc.).

Never go beyond the limits of what you are trained to do (i.e., only do Chiropractic adjustments if you are a Chiropractor, only do massage if you are trained in massage, and never do counseling unless you are trained in counseling).

Never touch anyone inappropriately.

Never take advantage of the bond that develops between you and the person you are treating. If you are treating someone in a therapeutic setting, it is inappropriate to date or have sexual relations with that person.

Respect the confidentiality of information given to you by your Reiki clients.

Never give away the Reiki. Dr. Usui said it makes beggars of the people you give it to. Remember, though, that the exchange can take many forms.

Be honest and accurate in the way you present yourself to the public regarding your level of Reiki training and other training and/or licensure.

It is not your responsibility to heal the world. You do not have to treat everyone. If it doesn't feel right to treat someone, don't do it.

Common sense should always be used when doing Reiki.

Disrobing is NOT necessary for a Reiki treatment. Do not have your client disrobe unless you are doing something in addition to Reiki, such as massage (and then only if you are licensed).

You should be fully clothed, and your clothing should be appropriate when doing a treatment. Many Reiki people prefer all-natural fibers because they tend to absorb any perspiration created.

> In caring for others and serving heaven,
> There is nothing like using restraint.
> Restraint begins with giving up one's own ideas.
> This depends on Virtue gathered in the past.
> If there is a good store of Virtue, then nothing is impossible.
> If nothing is impossible, then there are no limits.
> If a man knows no limits, then he is fit to be a ruler.
> The mother principle of ruling holds good for a long time.
> This is called having deep roots and a firm foundation,
> The Tao of long life and eternal vision.
>
> Lao Tsu
> —Tao Te Ching

Reiki is accepted or rejected at the soul level of the receiver. Your job is to be there; the rest is up to them. This holds true for whatever level of Reiki you are working with.

Reiki is simple; keep it that way. Don't let your ego make you think YOU are doing the healing. **Reiki does the healing.**

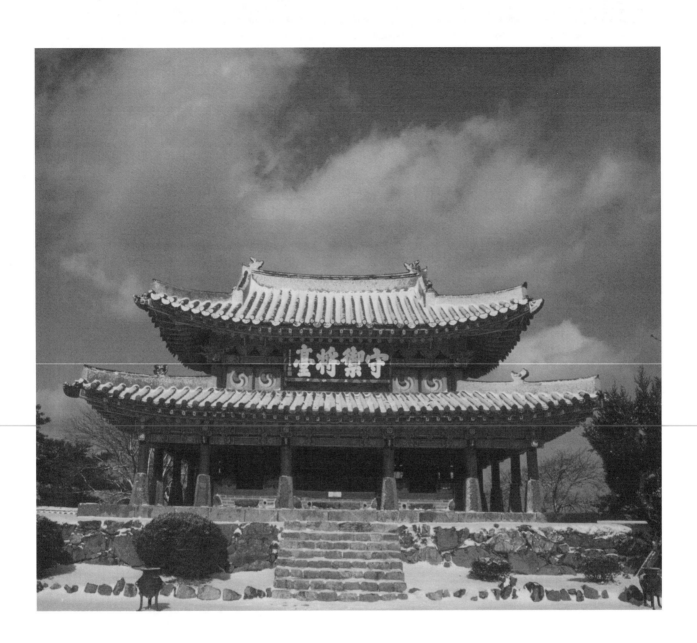

The Reiki Center

The purpose of the Reiki Center is twofold: its first purpose is to be a support organization for Reiki therapists. For those looking for a band-aid, Reiki is a great one. It will fix all those little "owies" of life, both physically and emotionally, and work on many of the serious physical ailments as well. For those looking for a tool of personal transformation, Reiki is the finest one I have ever found. Transformation can be a process that is best done in a supportive loving atmosphere, and that is where our Reiki Center comes in.

The Center's second purpose is to educate the public about Reiki. My original message was to make Reiki a household word in California. I have done my best to accomplish this goal. Wearing my hat as Director of the Reiki Center, I have spoken at many conferences and Expos, not just in California, but in other states across the country.

The Center had an unlikely beginning.

In the early '80s I was living in Dayton, Ohio and commuting to California to teach Reiki. On one of my trips I walked into a space and this little voice said, "This would make a great Reiki Center." I was startled and thought that was the craziest idea in the world, since I lived in Ohio and had no intention of starting a center anywhere other than where I lived. Not only that, but I was not financially in a position to support a center, nor did I have the time or the energy needed to support a center, and certainly not in a place I did not live, and where I had no intention of living.

> Come to the edge, he said.
> They said: We are afraid.
> Come to the edge, he said.
> They came.
> He pushed them
>   ... and they flew.
>
> Guillaume Apollinaire

I learned a long time ago about the "whispers" from the Universe. You know the ones I mean: first come the whispers; if you don't listen to them, next come the screams; if you still don't listen, next comes the 2x4 in whatever place is most effective. I really do try to listen to those whispers, because I don't like the screams and I REALLY don't like the 2x4's. I signed the lease on our first Reiki Center. The Universe had what it wanted, as usual. Somehow that always happens when you are open to higher guidance. We now had a physical location in which to hold our classes, and a place to start holding Healing Nights. And so began our Monday and Thursday Healing Nights, a time of sharing, growth, healing, and companionship.

Even though I lived in Ohio, the Center thrived due to the efforts of our volunteers, dedicated practitioners who saw the effect of Reiki in their lives who wanted to maximize its effect and to share this prize with others. The glue that held it all together was provided by my sons Will and Michael. Together they handled all aspects of the Center when I was not in town, including supervising "work traders" who did work in exchange for their training (we have never had to turn anyone away for lack of funds). And so the Reiki Center grew.

In the early days of the Center we succeeded in becoming both a Federal and a State Non-Profit Corporation. I have been told we were the first such organization based totally on the needs of the practitioners and the education of the public.

The Reiki Center continues to grow and evolve as our Reiki family continues to grow and evolve. Our current form has always been and still is to have a physical location in the Los Angeles area, and to have Healing

Nights in the other areas where we teach. At the center we have weekly Healing Nights for all our therapists, and a separate advanced healing night for our Second Degree Therapists only. Frequently the group goes out to a local cafe for socializing afterwards.

We also periodically have various social and spiritual activities, an annual daylong workshop on Creating a Spiritual Foundation for Prosperity, free Reiki workshops, and trainings on all three levels of Reiki. Our support groups meet in therapist's homes, metaphysical centers, and bookstores for Healing Nights and social functions throughout the country.

The dream has always been to have not only the main Center in Los Angeles, but also to have satellite Centers in a variety of areas and one or more Retreat Centers. These have not manifested as yet, but one never knows what is on the horizon when Reiki is involved. My experience has been, "What Reiki wants, Reiki gets." I have seen this hold true so many times, in so many ways. We have grown through four different physical Reiki Centers so far. It will be interesting to see what the Universe has in store for us in the future.

Every moment of your life
is infinitely creative
and the universe
is endlessly bountiful.

Just put forth
a clear enough request,
and everything
your heart desires
must come to you.

Shakti Gawain

The Three Degrees

In Oriental spiritual practices and martial arts, knowledge is divided into degrees based on a person's skill, abilities, and potential. As the person learns the lessons and develops the skills of one level, he or she progresses to the next level of knowledge, until the person reaches the highest potential. As an example, basic Tai Chi may work for everyone, intermediate level may work for some but not for others, and continuing on to become a teacher is for only a few. In a similar way, the lessons and skills of Reiki are divided into degrees.

FIRST DEGREE REIKI

First Degree Reiki is a method of hands-on treatment of yourself or others. This is the first step in a wonderful adventure that can be used to transform your life. Reiki brings balance, and as we become balanced, our bodies and psyches can heal themselves.

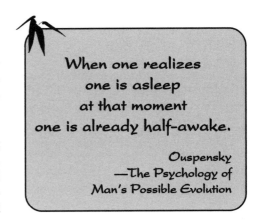

When one realizes
one is asleep
at that moment
one is already half-awake.

Ouspensky
—The Psychology of
Man's Possible Evolution

Four attunements tap you into this powerful method of healing at the First Degree. Once you have Reiki, you always have Reiki. You never lose it unless you choose to do something that would be in conflict with the Reiki energy. First Degree is a very powerful level of Reiki which is responsible for many of our "Reiki Miracle" stories.

Once you have been attuned to the Reiki energy, the only thing you have to do to turn it on is to touch. Intent has nothing to do with activating or using this level of Reiki. That is why even babies can be attuned to the energy. I have attuned numerous children to Reiki, the youngest being 1-1/2 hours old. Reiki gives even infants the ability to heal themselves and others. Babies and children just naturally touch, especially if something hurts.

My personal belief is that we come into this life with a purpose. As we grow, we become more involved in the material world. When we begin to communicate by talking, at 18 months to 2 years, we frequently become more and more distracted from our "mission" and we tend to lose our connection to our source. I feel that many of the children coming onto the planet today are very special people, and I also feel that by having Reiki at an early age they will be able to stay more focused, in better communication with their source. By having the gift of healing themselves and others, they will be able to have more of an impact on the planet.

In your First Degree class you will learn the history of Reiki, what Reiki will and will not do, and the hand positions for treating yourself and others. You will get many different experiences of Reiki, including treatments on yourself and others. Remember, all the information you receive from your Master and from books is just the package that Reiki is wrapped in. Reiki is not a "mind thing." The limitations of language make it impossible to adequately explain how Reiki works. The ATTUNEMENTS are what give you Reiki. These attunements align your Crown, Third Eye, Throat, and Heart chakras, and minor chakras in the palms of your hands, as well as working on the electromagnetic field of the body.

Once it is sealed in during the final attunement of First Degree, Reiki will never leave you unless you attempt to teach Reiki when you have not been initiated as a teacher in the direct line of Dr. Usui, or you choose to receive initiation into another healing modality that is not in keeping with Reiki. I have found Reiki totally compatible with other ancient healing modalities learned by initiation, as well as those learned with the conscious mind. It is only through newer "channelled" or "mixed" techniques that I have seen people lose their Reiki, and of course it is always by choice that one gets these other initiations.

The more you use Reiki the stronger it gets and the more it becomes part of your life.

SECOND DEGREE REIKI

Second Degree builds on the foundation laid with the 4 attunements of First Degree. Second Degree is many orders of magnitude more powerful than First Degree and allows you to heal both in person and at a distance. In addition to these physical healings, Second Degree allows you to do special treatments on mental, emotional, and addictive problems. Whether giving Reiki in person or absentee, you are offering healing energy, and are in no way controlling another individual. Reiki cannot be used for the manipulation of others, only to bring harmony and balance.

Some of the sacred knowledge of Reiki is imparted to you at this level, and you are taught how to use it for manifestation purposes. Where the attunements of First Degree aligned you, the Second Degree attunement empowers you; it gives you the ability to use symbols and other sacred knowledge you receive.

We used to believe that 90 days were needed between First and Second Degree for a person to grow in the use of, and comfort with, the energy. We now know that the timing is much more personal than that. Some people need no delay, while some need 90 days, or 3 years, or 5 lifetimes. Inner knowing tells you when you are ready for the jump from First to Second Degree.

Second Degree is a major tool in the transformational process for those on an accelerated spiritual path. It can also be used for planetary and personal issues.

MASTER LEVEL or THIRD DEGREE REIKI

Originally Mastership was only for those dedicated to teaching Reiki. As the knowledge and practice of Reiki became more widespread, more and more people became interested in going beyond the Second Degree, although they knew that they would probably never be chosen to become Masters. At that time, in the mid-1980s, the Master level was divided into two parts. This allowed many to have some of this advanced knowledge for their own personal growth and development.

The first, or Master Therapist level (originally called "3A for Personal Growth"), is for those who are deeply spiritual and dedicated to service to Reiki. As Second Degree has orders of magnitude more powerful than First Degree, the Master level is infinitely more powerful than Second Degree. The initiation for Master Therapist activates to a broader and deeper level of healing energy. The primary reason most people go to this level is to be able to use the temporary activations or "Booster" attunements on themselves, others, and on planetary situations. At the Reiki Center we require a minimum of one year of working with the Second Degree energy before one can petition to be accepted for this advanced level of study. We consider this to be a level for service to Reiki, not something for ego inflation or power trips (more people are turned down for this level than are accepted). It is considered quite an honor to be able to serve Reiki in this way.

Master Teacher is the final level of Reiki Mastership. It is for those dedicated to teaching Reiki and to devoting their lives to Reiki. Masters are fully trained in the activations of First and Second Degree practitioners. The

Master initiation and an extensive apprenticeship allow new Master Teachers to teach, knowing that they are working with the true Reiki energy in as pure a form as possible.

A minimum of one year working with the Master Therapist energy is required before the initiating Master would consider a possible candidate for this level. At this level one is chosen, as has been practiced in Oriental systems for centuries.

> We therefore arrive
> at the principle
> that those interested
> in the prevention or cure
> of disease
> should have a knowledge
> of all gross and subtle
> aspects of the body.
> These range from the body,
> which is the end-organ
> of the nervous system,
> to the mind,
> which in turn extends
> from gross to subtle levels
> of thinking
> and touches
> the field of Being.
>
> Maharishi Mahesh Yogi

Begin difficult things
　while they are easy,

Do great things
　when they are small.

The difficult things of the world
　must once have been easy,

The great things
　must once have been small ...

A thousand mile journey
　begins with
　　one step.

Lao-Tse
—The Simple Way

Treatment Guidelines

You cannot harm yourself or others with Reiki, and you cannot do Reiki incorrectly (however, it is possible to do Reiki illegally, so do not touch in any inappropriate places). Remember that a little Reiki is better than no Reiki, and there is no such thing as too much Reiki.

A Reiki treatment will balance every organ, gland, chakra, and energy meridian. It therefore makes no difference if a person's beliefs are Eastern or Western; Reiki treats it all and brings every aspect of a person's life into a better state of balance.

With Reiki it is not necessary to stay focused on the healing process; such focusing can, however, make for a very powerful healing session. Reiki can be effective even when the practitioner or the client is talking, laughing, crying, making out a mental grocery list, sleeping or doing anything else. We are channels for the energy. It flows through us, and it is only dependent upon us for touch, not for focus.

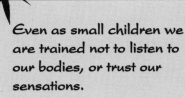

Even as small children we are trained not to listen to our bodies, or trust our sensations.

Gay Gaer Luce

Certain procedures are recommended when doing Reiki treatments:

- Treat yourself DAILY. As long as you treat all positions within a 24-hour period it counts as one treatment. Doing a full treatment at one sitting feels great, but fits into few people's schedules.

- I have found that using what is called Pacing and Leading can be very helpful when giving treatments. Start out by breathing at whatever pace your client is breathing. Very slowly start to change your own breathing pattern to a slow, rhythmic pace as you lead your client into changing his or her breathing pattern along with you. This helps to get the client relaxed more quickly, and helps to put the two of you onto the same wave length.

- Treat in each position until you feel the "rise and fall of energy," or, if you do not have a physical experience of the energy, just treat for 5 minutes.

During the "rise," or build-up of energy, you may feel a variety of sensations. These could be heat, cold, tingling, throbbing, the sensation of your hand being pushed up as if a balloon is under it, or as if your hand is being drawn down inside the person's body—or none. All are simply manifestations of the Reiki energy. The "fall" of energy is when the sensation you are feeling changes. That is your sign that it is time to move on to the next position.

- If you cannot treat directly on the body, you may treat the auric field, 1 to 5 inches from the body. This is especially helpful in treating burns or contagious skin diseases, or when you must treat through a cast.

- Reiki will go through cloth, leather, or almost anything, including the cast on a broken arm or leg. It is wise, however, to remove rubber-soled shoes because the sensations of the energy are diminished for the recipient.

The traditional method for maximum healing results is to give full treatments on 3 or 4 consecutive days. My preferred protocol is a series of 10 treatments in the first month: 3 or 4 in the first week, 3 in the second week, 2 in the third week, 1 in the fourth week, and then as needed, usually monthly.

In critical situations, it was not unusual for Madam Takata to physically move in with the family, in order to give lengthy daily treatments. She also frequently required that all family members receive the initiations. This meant that the client would be surrounded with the Reiki energy 24 hours a day.

- Wash your hands before and after giving a treatment. If this is impossible, place the fingertips together for a few seconds to break the energy flow after treatment. We do this to avoid inadvertently transferring energy from one client to another and to break the flow between practitioner and client.

- To ensure the free flow of energy, be sure the client does not cross his or her legs during the treatment. Also make sure the client removes tight belts, glasses, shoes, and jewelry.

- Place a pillow under the client's knees to ease any strain on the back and place a pillow under the head for comfort.

- Have a blanket at hand, for the body temperature drops after reclining for a few minutes.

- A massage table tends to be the most comfortable place to give a treatment; however, any place will do: sofa cushions on a dining room table or the floor, the end of a bed with a chair for the therapist, a chair for the client with the therapist standing or sitting, etc. Remember, for both you and the client: **COMFORT, COMFORT, COMFORT.**

- With the flow of energy, clients often experience an emotional release, so keep tissues handy.

- Place a tissue over the client's eyes, folded as a triangle, with the point towards the top of their head.

- Let your client know that a Reiki treatment does not end with the Reiki Finish. The energy will continue to flow for 24 to 48 hours. People who are sensitive to energy may experience changes during that time.

Certain issues need to be addressed when doing Reiki treatments:

- NEVER diagnose or prescribe unless you are licensed to do so.

- Be fastidious with your personal hygiene. When giving a treatment you are extremely close to your client, so be sure you are not offensive in any way, and make sure you don't use anything that could cause an allergic reaction.

- Use no perfumes or aftershaves because of possible chemical sensitivities or allergies. Often in illness the sense of smell is more acute, so even mild fragrances may be disturbing to your client.

- Keep your fingers **gently** together during a treatment. Mme. Takata said, **"Scattered fingers are scattered energy."**

- You can talk during a treatment; it will not diminish what you are doing, but remember to let the client set the pace. It's the client's time, and not yours.

- Rest your hands lightly during the treatment; heavy hands are not comfortable to your client. It is especially important to never put pressure on the client's **eyes** or **throat**.

- Hands should touch on the midline of the body to assure that the endocrine glands and spinal cord nerves are treated.

- Cleanse the room both before and after giving a treatment. I like to use incense in combination with the 2nd Degree cleansing technique; however you may use sage, essential oils, or the cleansing technique by itself. Be sure to use incense prepared by a spiritual group so that it gives off a high vibration.

- Never say Reiki "cures." It is best to say that it balances, that it allows the body to heal itself, that it harmonizes, etc. Never give anyone false hope, and never give a prognosis. Remember we never know on what level or in what time frame Reiki will work with any particular individual.

- Reiki dislodges toxins and buildups throughout your body, so remember the importance of both therapist and client drinking lots of water to flush the toxins out of the system. Toxins which are not quickly flushed out will be re-absorbed into the body.

- Reiki balances and heals "phantom organs" (surgically removed) just as it would a "phantom limb." For this reason you may still feel a strong rise and fall of energy where there is no physical organ (e.g., tonsils, uterus, etc.).

Reiki is great as a preventive treatment. It helps you or your client to reach a state of optimal health and balance. When in a balanced state few dis-eases can take hold.

When you give Reiki, remember that the energy fills you up before it flows out from your hands. Therefore, you receive a treatment in the process of giving one. Truly with Reiki **as you give, so shall ye receive."**

Through faith, anything is possible. My faith in the presence of God within me is sufficient to heal, to adjust in harmony, and to move a mountain of challenge that is before me.

Daily Word
(Association of Unity Churches)

To hate another is to hate yourself,
We all live within the one
    Universal Mind.
What we think about another,
we think about ourselves.

If you have an enemy, forgive him
    now.
Let all bitterness and resentment
    dissolve.
You owe your fellow man love,
show him love, not hate.

Show charity and goodwill toward
    others
and it will return to enhance
your own life
in many wonderful ways.

Brian Adams
—How to Succeed

Team Treatments

Whenever more than one person treats at the same time with Reiki, there is an exponential increase in the healing energy. In other words, if six people are treating, it is not 6 times the energy of one, but rather a minimum of 6 squared and possibly as high as 6 to the 10th power. This exponential increase is why our healing support groups that meet on a regular basis have such wonderful outcomes from their work.

When doing team treatments, the head and torso are the primary areas to be treated. If there are enough people treating, then treating the feet runs energy through the reflex areas on the soles of the feet up into all areas of the body. And of course if there is a problem area, be sure to treat it after the head and torso have been treated.

An ideal team treatment would be to have one person treating the head, two on each side of the torso, one on each side of the legs (each treating a knee and an ankle), and one treating the feet. If there are extra people, they can place their hands on someone seated at the table treating the client.

Legal Considerations

I am asked frequently what one needs to do to have a Reiki practice. There is no one answer to this question because it depends on the legal requirements of the place you want to practice. When you finish a Reiki class you get a certificate. That is totally different from getting a license to charge money for treatment sessions. Licenses are given primarily by governmental bodies: states, counties or townships, and cities. What is legal on one side of the street could be illegal on the other side of the street if it is in a different jurisdiction.

It is very important for you to be legal if you are going to work on the public and charge a fee. If you are giving treatments to your family and friends, the legal requirements are looser; besides, of course, general decency and the patient's consent. If, however, you wish to work on the public, make sure you abide by whatever laws are in force in the area in which you wish to practice. Local regulations and information are available at your City Hall. Be aware, however, that you may end up getting investigated by the Vice Squad, as they are usually responsible for regulating hands-on treatment.

One of the reasons I feel it necessary to have a new workbook is that many of the hand positions shown in previous workbooks are illegal. They show the therapist's hands on both the breasts and genitals and on bare skin. In the Orient where Reiki originated, the laws regarding where you can place your hands on another person are quite different from the laws in the United States. We try to keep the Reiki technique pure, however it is extremely important that when doing Reiki you are **totally legal and ethical in all that you do at all times.** This is far more important than abiding by the hand positions we were taught years ago.

He who stands on tiptoe is not steady.
He who strides cannot maintain the pace.
He who makes a show is not enlightened.
He who is self-righteous is not respected.
He who boasts achieves nothing.
He who brags will not endure.
According to followers of the Tao,
    "These are extra food and unnecessary
        luggage."
They do not bring happiness.
Therefore followers of the Tao avoid them.

Lao Tsu
—Tao Te Ching

The Temptations

If you are on a spiritual path you WILL be tempted. That is part of spiritual growth. The temptations are there for you to overcome and grow by, not to be hung up in and wallow in. You will also be tempted by what you are most temptable with: if hot fudge sundaes are your weakness, you won't be tempted with spinach salad. Whatever temptations you have already worked through will not need to come up for you again in this lifetime, unless of course there are other and probably deeper levels yet to be conquered. So what you will find is that when you are least expecting it, up will pop one of these green-headed monsters. Reiki often accelerates this process.

At this time, it is wise to have a few friends you can count on who are willing to be totally, and some might even say brutally, honest. When you are being challenged by one of the temptations you will almost assuredly not be able to see it for yourself. This is when you will need your friends, willing and able to confront you about the issue. Confront is what your friend will probably have to do, because what you are into will seem absolutely right to you. What are these green-headed monsters I call THE TEMPTATIONS?

Pride

Ego

Greed

"Power Hungriness"

Awareness that you WILL be tempted, be it now or later, makes it easier on a daily basis to really look at what is going on in your life. Students usually ask what the specific temptations will be once they start on a Reiki path. The temptations will show up in all areas of your life; with respect to Reiki, usually they will have something to do with wanting to be a Reiki Master, or with thinking YOU are doing the healing rather than the Reiki energy doing the healing.

> **Pride** might make you want the title of Reiki Master and think that you, not your Master, are the one to decide this.
>
> **Ego** might make you feel you have "earned" or that you "deserve" the right to be a Reiki Master. Or that YOU, not Reiki, is doing the the healing.
>
> **Greed** might lead you to believe you can be a Reiki Master for less than the $10,000 Dr. Hayashi set as its value.
>
> **Power Hungriness** might make you think you should have power over other humans, and be stronger in your Reiki than they are.

You should also be aware that the "higher" you go on a spiritual path the harder the lessons get. Some think the lessons should get easier, but they do not: **beginners get beginning lessons, advanced students get advanced lessons.** That is how we grow. Remember that we all have free will and are never forced into any growth we don't want. Reiki supports and assists growth, but we can still always get off the bandwagon at any time we wish. It's totally up to us.

What we do today
creates our future,
as the shadow follows the body
so we are followed
by the law of fate.
Each is forced to bear
the consequences of his actions
himself.

Padma-Sambhava

Inner peace
can be reached
only when we practice
forgiveness.

Forgiveness
is the letting go of the past,
and is therefore the means
for correcting
our misperceptions.

Gerald G. Jampolsky
—Love is Letting Go of Fear

Transformation Tools

Reiki is without a doubt the finest tool for transformation I have ever found. People who are actively involved in their spiritual development will be amazed at what Reiki will do **"in, through, and as you."** Why spend five lifetimes working through or learning something when you can do it in five years? Why spend five years when it can be accomplished in five minutes? With Reiki you will definitely be on that fast track.

Many changes will take place in the days and months after taking Reiki. I strongly recommend you start keeping a journal; consciously recognizing the before and after comparisons can be very exciting.

We have many other tools available to us that can be used in conjunction with Reiki to speed up and/or facilitate the growth and transformational process. I want to share with you some of the tools I have used and that I have found to be the most beneficial. My hope is that you can use this information in your growth process. I do not believe that we must constantly reinvent the wheel. We can learn from others, from their triumphs and their failures. To do this we must keep an open mind, be very observant, and be willing to risk.[1]

DETOX AND PURIFICATION

In order to be in peak physical and mental condition many people feel that detoxification and purification are important. Some students are led to do cleansing and purification rites before taking Reiki. This is not required, or even necessary, though it can be excellent for some people. You will know if it is right for you.

Detoxing, however, does occur while you are in class and going through the attunements, and while treating yourself and others—and it continues for quite some time afterwards. Remember to keep drinking water to flush these toxins out of your system.

Deep breathing is a wonderful tool of detox, because the lungs are the second largest organ of detox in the body, second only to the skin. If you are not familiar with deep breathing or yoga breathing techniques, find yourself a good yoga teacher and start TODAY.

Many alternative healing modalities include the concept of a "Healing Crisis." Chiropractic treatments, massage, homeopathic healings, nutritional therapies, specialized diets, Reiki, and many other techniques can "trigger" a healing crisis. This is a process of going from the chronic phase of a challenge back through the acute phase, as old symptoms may come to the surface to be released on the way to good health. As long as we have dis-ease in cellular memory it will continue to be a time bomb waiting to cause problems. By releasing these traumas from cellular memory, true healing can occur. With Reiki this clearing can take place on the physical, mental, emotional or spiritual levels. Madam Takata said it usually takes from 4 days to 3 weeks for this "purging" or "reacting" process.

> Life is full
> and overflowing
> with the new.
>
> But it is necessary
> to empty out the old
> to make room for
> the new to enter.
>
> Eileen Caddy
> —Footprints on the Path

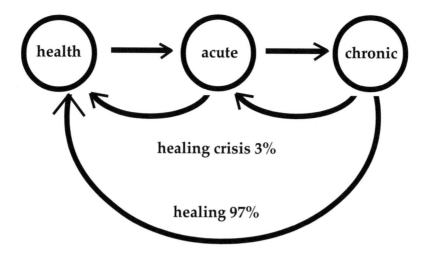

health → acute → chronic

healing crisis 3%

healing 97%

Epsom Salt baths are a very old technique to speed up the removal of water-soluble toxins from the body. I use a full box, 4 pounds, of Epsom Salts in a very hot tub, as hot as I can take it, for a minimum of 20 minutes and a maximum of 30 minutes. I then shower the residue off, get into bed, and sleep like an angel. The next morning I feel wonderful, and find that any cold or flu symptoms, or emotional upsets, are a thing of the past.

Many excellent books are available to guide you through a detoxing process if you choose to speed it up. I personally like the Edgar Cayce apple fast,[2] and I use it at the change of seasons and at other times I feel I would like to detox and cleanse, be it physically or emotionally. This is a short, 3 day process. Other programs may be shorter or longer, rigorous or simple. Experiment to find out what works best for you. Two recipes handed down to us as traditional Reiki cleansing tools are given at the end of this section (page 63).

PRAYER

Prayer is talking to God, or Goddess, or Higher Power, or whatever word is right for YOU—not what was right for your parents, your friends, or anyone else but you. As you get into closer communication with your Higher Power (let's just use the word God—it's so much easier), you will find that your prayer time and your meditation time become a vital part of every day, and that without this special time you will feel a loss.

Prayer is not always "asking for," although it certainly can be at times. Prayer can also be sharing what your day has been like, asking for guidance and focus in your life. Certainly "thanksgiving" is also a vital part of most people's prayer life. When you have "thanksgiving" as an integral part of every day you will find more things manifesting in your life to give thanks for.

> What things soever ye desire,
> when ye pray,
> Believe that ye receive them,
> and ye shall have them.
>
> Mark 11:24
> —King James Bible

If you have never prayed, a good way to start is to just pretend you are talking to your best friend. Tell that friend what's going on with you, what you are happy about, what is bothering you. If it makes it easier, use a different name other than God. One friend of mine called God "Pop," because it neutralized all her old training as to who and what God was (an old white man standing on a cloud, in a long white gown and white beard, scolding her and telling her how bad she was).

Remember prayer and meditation, when used together, are powerful transformational tools—they will change your life.

MEDITATION

Meditation is a major tool for growth and transformation. I consider that prayer is talking to God, and meditation is listening to the answers, or the guidance. These answers can come in many ways—sometimes from a billboard as we drive down the highway, or from a song on the radio as we "happen" to turn it on, perhaps from a chance comment we overhear in someone else's conversation, or from a dream. The sources are endless—but we must be listening.

There is no one right way to meditate. There are many forms of meditation and, again, you must find out which one or ones are best for you. You may find that you like to use several different modalities depending on your mood of the day, the amount of time you have to devote to your meditation that day, your level of privacy, etc. Many people find that 2 short meditations each day of 15 or 20 minutes rather than one long meditation can be quite transformational. Even five minutes spent in meditation can shift the energy of your day.

Often people find it difficult to begin meditating on their own, alone. For this reason I strongly recommend taking a meditation class to get started. To find a class, check out your local metaphysical bookstores, New Thought churches in your area, the TM (Transcendental Meditation)[3] Center, Self Realization Fellowship,[4] or Yoga Centers near you. Meditation has become so widely practiced that there are often classes at the local YMCA or YWCA or at local community colleges.[5]

> If you cannot compose yourself to thought continually, then compose yourself from time to time, at least twice a day, in the morning and the evening. In the morning form your resolution, and in the evening consider how you have conducted yourself today in thought, word, and deed.
>
> Thomas a Kempis
> —Imitatio Christi

EXERCISES:

General Instructions—
Take the phone off the hook or turn the ringer off.
Get comfortable in a chair or on the floor.
Have a blanket handy (body temperature will drop).
Create a healing environment—lights, music, etc.
Take a few seconds to get centered.
Do deep, slow breathing to relax.
Begin with 10 minutes and build up to 20 minutes.

Candle Meditation—
Place a candle where it will be safe, easily visible and not in a draft.
Have the room dark except for the burning candle.
Stare at the candle and become one with the flame.

Chanting—
Choose a word or words that you are comfortable with and repeat them over and over again in your head, or out loud, until they become a part of you.
Some of the single words most used are AUM or OM, AMEN, and ALLELUIA.
Some longer chants that have been used for centuries are OM NAMAHA SHIVAYA, OM SHIVA, THY WILL BE DONE, and THE LORD'S PRAYER. Most religions have their own prayers or words that can be used as chants.

White Light Meditation—
Imagine a beautiful cloud over your head.
Slowly the cloud opens up and out streams a beautiful WHITE LIGHT that flows down and around you, totally surrounding you with its warmth and comfort.
Affirm—I am surrounded by the WHITE LIGHT of Health, Peace, Prosperity, Love, Mental, Physical and Spiritual well being, no harm can enter in, Divine Right Order.
Continue basking in the light until it permeates every cell of your being.

POSITIVE THOUGHT & AFFIRMATIONS

I have been a student of Positive Thought work[6] for many years and have found it can be enhanced when used in conjunction with Reiki treatments, especially over the heart and the first three head positions. We each have within us an internal voice, and for most people this voice talks to us in a rather constant, negative manner. To change this negative thought process into a positive one usually takes effort, but it can be done. Listening to positive thought tapes, reading positive thought books and surrounding yourself with positive rather than negative people **will make the difference.**

Release is part of this type of work, for we must release the negative to make room for the positive. It is another tool that can be used to facilitate the growth process, and can very effectively be used in conjunction with a detox program.[7] Reiki is especially helpful in speeding up the process of cleaning out the old to make way for the new. Working to release "what is" for "what can be" is sometimes frightening, always exciting, and definitely growth producing—for the "what can be" is always better than the "what is."

Throughout this workbook I have placed numerous affirmations from a wide variety of wonderful teachers, spiritual paths and books. I hope you enjoy them as much as I do.

> What we are today comes from our thoughts of yesterday, and our present thoughts build our life of tomorrow:
> Our life is the creation of our mind.
>
> The Buddha

EXERCISES:

Growth jar - put a quarter (or a dollar or a dime or whatever amount you decide you can afford by stretching it) into your jar whenever you say a negative word or think a negative thought.

Create a tape, in your own voice, of positive affirmations that are especially pertinent for you. Listen to it while driving, sleeping, or doing repetitive tasks.

Put affirmations around your home, office, and car. Put them inside cupboard doors and medicine cabinets, on mirrors, on dash boards, etc.

GUIDED VISUALIZATION

To speed up your healing, growth, change and transformational process, many people use the technique of Guided Visualization. Wonderful books and tapes are available today to help you to create what you want in your life, whether that is improved health, increased prosperity, enhanced relationships, spiritual growth, or something else you might desire.[8] Try some of these tapes, or create your own tapes from the material you find in the books. Be very cautious about creating your own affirmations and visualizations; it is very easy to create the opposite of what you desire by using the wrong wording.

When I was a full-time counselor I created a series of guided visualizations for use with my clients. The most effective visualizations are being made into a series of audiotapes; the first three are currently available. For healing needs I have gotten wonderful feedback about my Color Breathing tape. It has been used effectively in both "pre-op" and "post-op" situations, and for insomnia. For clearing and purification, the Water Purification tape is extremely effective, and for spiritual growth try Getting In Touch with Your Higher Self. These are only a few of the wonderful tapes currently available to you.

I have found that pillow speakers (available at Radio Shack) used with auto reverse tape players make excellent use of sleep time. Small personal cassette players with lightweight headphones can be used to make good use of the time spent doing repetitive tasks that don't require thinking. There just aren't enough hours in the day to accomplish all we would like to accomplish, so we have to be creative in how we do use our time. Remember what you put into your head is just as important, if not more important, than what you put into your mouth. The unconscious is more receptive during sleeptime, so be mindful about the resources you choose to use.

> Whatever you can do
> or dream you can,
> begin it.
>
> Boldness has genius, magic
> and power in it.
>
> Begin it now.
>
> Goethe

EXERCISES:
See "General Instructions" under the Meditation section.

ROSE VISUALIZATION
Start by doing slow, deep, uniform breathing.
Visualize a rose bud. See it in full detail and color.
Very, very slowly see the bud start to open.
Savor each movement as the bud grows into full bloom.
Watch as each petal slowly drops to the ground.
Wonder at the growth of the rose hip filling with seeds.
Experience the joy as the rose hip explodes and sprays its seeds into the wind.
Feel the chill as the snow blankets the small seed.
Expand with the seed as it sends out roots into the ground.
Grow with the stem as it reaches for the light and the warmth of the sun.
Stretch with the leaves as they unfurl to soak up the sun.
Feel the bud start to form as another season begins.

BREATHING

In our culture we are usually taught from the time we are small to "stand up straight, pull in your tummy and tuck in your butt." The result is that we only breathe with the upper part of our lungs and never learn to breathe deeply. This is not a healthy habit, so most of us need to learn to do deep breathing or Yoga breathing as it is sometimes called.

Although there are no specific breathing rituals connected with Reiki, treating yourself or another while working with various breathing techniques can be very helpful and empowering.

EXERCISES:

Color Breathing
Breathe in a soft healing color.
See the color swirl throughout your body melting any tension or dis-ease. As it picks up the melted "gunk" it will become dark and muddy.
Allow the "gunk" to flow out your feet making puddles on the floor.
See the puddles transmuted as they flow into a beautiful violet flame.
When the color coming out your feet is the same as the color you are breathing in, the healing cycle will be complete.

Alternate Nostril Breathing
Place the thumb of your right hand on your right nostril, your 1st and 2nd fingers between the eyebrows, and your ring finger on the left nostril.
Hold the right nostril shut, breathe in for a count of 4.
Hold both nostrils shut for a count of 4.
Breathe out through the left nostril for a count of 4.
Hold both nostrils shut for a count of 4.
Hold the left nostril shut, breathe in for a count of 4.
Hold both nostrils shut for a count of 4.
Breathe out through the right nostril for a count of 4.
Hold both nostrils shut for a count of 4.

Repeat for approximately 10 minutes. This technique is especially useful as a preparation for meditating.
Instead of a count of 4-4-4, you can use 6-6-6 , 4-6-4 or 6-8-6 or any other count that feels good to you.

TWELVE STEP PROGRAMS

Probably the most widely known (other than prayer) of the many Tools for Transformation is Alcoholics Anonymous.[9] Because of its success rate there are numerous "Anonymous" programs using the same steps, such as Overeaters, Gamblers, Narcotics, Debtors, Al-Anon, Codependents, Adult Children of Alcoholics, Sexual Addicts and Emotional Health.

AA was formed when two men, Dr. Bob and Bill W., joined together to help each other recover from the disease of alcoholism. Their 12-step program of recovery has been used by thousands of people world wide and has offered strength and hope to those in need. These same 12 steps can be used by anyone seeking to transform their lives and find a spiritual foundation for life. Among the numerous 12-step programs I'm sure you will find one or more that meet your needs.

To locate AA or another type of 12-step program near you check in the yellow pages of the telephone book under "associations," or in the white pages under the actual name. Here are the 12 steps of AA as given in chapter 5 of the Big Book of Alcoholics Anonymous:

> Often the one thing we really want to do in life is not begun because of the fear we feel just thinking about it. The greatest growth and personal development is achieved through taking a risk and facing those fears. The time you least feel like starting something is precisely the time to Begin It Now.
>
> Susan Hayward
> —Begin it Now

60

The "12 STEPS" - "How it Works," chapter 5, of the BIG BOOK of AA

1. We admitted we were powerless over alcohol—that our lives had become unmanageable.
2. Came to believe that a Power greater than ourselves could restore us to sanity.
3. Made a decision to turn our will and our lives over to the care of God as we understood Him.
4. Made a searching and fearless moral inventory of ourselves.
5. Admitted to God, to ourselves, and to another human being the exact nature of our wrongs.
6. Were entirely ready to have God remove all these defects of character.
7. Humbly asked Him to remove our shortcomings.
8. Made a list of all persons we had harmed, and became willing to make amends to them all.
9. Made direct amends to such people whenever possible, except when to do so would injure them or others.
10. Continued to take personal inventory, and when we were wrong, promptly admitted it.
11. Sought through prayer and meditation to improve our conscious contact with God *as we understood Him* praying only for knowledge of His will for us and the power to carry that out.
12. Having had a spiritual experience as the result of these steps, we tried to carry this message to alcoholics, and to practice these principles in all our affairs.[10]

The Steps of AA incorporate many of the tools for transformation that we are discussing in other sections, such as detoxing, prayer and meditation, gratitude, and aligning oneself with divine guidance. As you can see, these are also very closely aligned with the Principles of Reiki given to us by Dr. Usui.

LIFE STYLE CHANGES

Reiki is not a "silver bullet" or a "fix all" system. It can, and often does, create massive change in health, prosperity, spiritual growth, relationships, etc. It works on them all. However, to maintain what Reiki creates you will probably find you must make changes in your life, or your lifestyle. These changes may be in the way you think (this is what I find most frequently in need of change), the food you eat, the words you speak, your addictions, your lifestyle and any number of other aspects of your life.[11]

Reiki can facilitate change, but if you do not work at the level of whatever created the problem in the first place, then chances are the problem will return. The problem isn't that Reiki didn't work, the problem is that you didn't. Have you noticed how many times "you" has come up in this section? Only you can make the changes in your life that will create the life that you want. I hope you have fun doing it and that this workbook will make your journey easier and more enjoyable.

> Evil thoughts are originators of disease, for every thought is a little hammer blow on the metal of our body and beats out what we shall be. We are the heirs of all good thoughts in the Universe if we open ourselves to them.
>
> Vivekananda

KARMA

Every culture has a concept of karma; they just call it by different names:

"An eye for an eye, a tooth for a tooth"

"What goes around comes around"

"Everyone gets their just deserts"

"The law of tenfold return"

"As you sow, so shall you reap"

The core truth in all of these is the law of cause and effect. Whatever we give out, we get back. If we give out joy, love and happiness, that is what we will get back; if we give out hatred, anger, and frustration, then that is what will come back to us. Sometimes we have "instant Karma" when what we give out comes back quickly; sometimes we have delayed karma when it waits months, years or even lifetimes before coming back; sometimes what we are going through are experiences or lessons that offer other people opportunities to work through their karma.

Dealing with our Karma in the present time is a true tool of transformation, because when we balance out our Karma we are no longer being held down by it. In Second Degree Reiki we have a technique to facilitate this process. The Karmic implications of our choices today matter in our life today, not just in our future reincarnations. Karmic ties with other individuals can hold us back or support us in our growth. By balancing these Karmic ties, we release the past, known or unknown, so that we may grow to our full potential in this lifetime.

Karma seems to be something that many people do not understand. As you progress on your spiritual path, it is important for you to realize the Karmic ramifications of your actions. I see many people going astray, even leading others astray, without giving any thought to the Karmic outcome. Look at Jonestown and Waco as prime examples. The Karmic implications of our daily decisions matter just as much. For more clarity refer to the books listed at the end of this chapter.[12]

Karma is not bad or good; it is only payment in kind for what you give out. Be very careful with what you give out, because you **WILL** get it back **tenfold.**

PROSPERITY

As a culture we tend to have many misconceptions regarding prosperity. Think for a moment of all the negative statements you have heard regarding money—"filthy rich," "money is the root of all evil," "gold-digger," "money hungry," etc. The list goes on and on. The truth is that, as with Karma, money is neither good nor bad. Money is simply a means of exchange, a handy tool for barter. It is much less messy to carry around money in your wallet than a cherry pie, but they both have a certain value and can be used to "pay" for something. Part of spiritual growth is learning to put this into perspective.

You are all LIGHT BEARERS or you would not be studying something like Reiki. It is extremely important that as light bearers you improve your prosperity consciousness and overcome any beliefs you might have in lack and limitation. If you must work 10 to 14 hours a day to just barely earn enough money to put food on the table and a roof over your head, then there will not be enough money to buy the books you need to study for spiritual growth and development, or the time to read them. Nor will you have the money to study with the teachers you are ready to learn from, wherever they may be in the world. It is also very important for you to financially and emotionally support the things you believe in, for if you don't, who will? And more importantly, you will not have the time to share this knowledge with others on a spiritual path.

Prosperous thinking is something that is part of some people's upbringing. In most families, however, the training seems to focus more on lack and limitation. Many wonderful books and seminars are available for helping you change into a more positive, prosperous person. Catherine Ponder's book, *Open Your Mind to Prosperity*, should be required reading for all people on a spiritual path, and I recommend it for all of my Second Degree students.

God is my source!
My good is coming
to me now!

Daily Word
(Association of
Unity Churches)

At the first of each year I teach a very special day-long workshop on "How to Create a Spiritual Foundation for Prosperity." This workshop is limited to our Second Degree Reiki people and requires

62

them to make a full year commitment to becoming prosperous. It consists of many exercises used throughout the year to assist in changing old thought patterns of lack and limitation into new ones of prosperity, success, health, and happiness. Many New Thought churches have similar seminars, so you might wish to check into one in your area.[13]

Reiki is a powerful tool for supporting oneself through the fear that comes with making changes in breaking down old beliefs, habits and behaviors. I truly do believe that Spirituality, Prosperity, and Good Health are all very closely related, and that to have one you must also have, or at least strive for, the others.

TRADITIONAL REIKI CLEANSING/DETOXING RECIPES

REIKI SLAW

1 head each cauliflower and cabbage, grated

3-4 large raw beets

5-6 stalks celery, finely chopped

1 or more onions , finely chopped

Mix thoroughly with the hands (to add Reiki energy). Add dressing of your choice. Eat one cup daily to keep the intestines functioning well.

BLOOD PURIFIER

1 large head white or green cabbage

1 large bunch watercress

3-4 raw beets

4-5 stalks celery

Blend thoroughly to a liquid consistency. Use for a week-long fast, drinking as much as desired. Remember to also drink ample water.

1. Kathy Mengle, *Tools for Healing: Working toward Harmony and Balance* (Marina del Rey, CA: DeVorss, 1987); and Ingrid S. Von Rohr, *Harmony is the Healer* (Boston: Element, 1992).
2. William McGarey, *The Edgar Cayce Remedies* (New York: Bantam, 1983); Herbert Puryear, *The Edgar Cayce Primer* (New York: Bantam, 1982); Reba A. Karp, *Edgar Cayce Encyclopedia of Healing* (New York: Warner, 1988).
3. Maharishi Vedic Schools, 1-888-LEARNTM or visit their web page at www.tm.org.
4. Self-Realization Fellowship, 17190 Sunset Blvd., Pacific Palisades, CA, 90272, (323) 225-2471.
5. Herbert Benson and Miriam Z. Klipper, *The Relaxation Response* (New York: Avon, 1976); Audio tape by Daniel Goleman, "The Art of Meditation" (Los Angeles: Audio Renaissance, 1989).
6. Catherine Ponder, *Open Your Mind to Prosperity*; and *The Prospering Power of Love*; and *The Healing Secrets of the Ages* (Marina Del Rey, CA: DeVorss, 1971, 1966, 1985); and *The Dynamic Laws of Healing* (Marina Del Rey, CA: DeVorss, 1966); and Florence Scovel Shinn, *The Wisdom of Florence Scovel Shinn* (New York: Simon & Schuster, 1989); Louise Hay, *You Can Heal Your Life* (Carson, CA: Hay House, 1984); Douglas Bloch, *Listening to Your Inner Voice* (Minneapolis, MN: CompCare, 1991); and *Words That Heal* (New York: Bantam, 1990); See also *Daily Word* and *Unity Magazine* (Association of Unity Churches).
7. Audio tape by Joyce J. Morris, "Healing I—Color Breathing and Affirmations" (Encino, CA: Reiki, 1990).
8. Jeanne Achterberg, Barbara Dossey, and Leslie Kolkmeier, *Rituals of Healing: Using Imagery for Health and Wellness* (New York: Bantam, 1994); Shakti Gawain, *Creative Visualization* (Mill Valley, CA: Nataraj, 1978); and *Living in the Light* (Mill Valley, CA: Nataraj Publishing, 1986); Audio tape by Brugh Joy, "Healing with Body Energy" (Los Angeles: Audio Renaissance Tapes, 1987); Serge King, *Imagineering for Health* (Wheaton, IL: Quest Books, 1991); William

Fezler, *Creative Imagery* (New York: Simon & Schuster, 1989); Audio tapes by Joyce J. Morris, "Healing II—Water Purification" (Encino, CA: Reiki, 1991); and "Getting In Touch With Your Higher Self" (Encino, CA: Reiki, 1990); see also Marilee Zdenek, *Inventing the Future: Advances in Imagery That Can Change Your Life* (New York: McGraw-Hill, 1987).

9. *Alcoholics Anonymous* (New York: Alcoholics Anonymous World Services, 1976, 3rd edition); and *Came to Believe* (New York: Alcoholics Anonymous World Services).

10. *Alcoholics Anonymous*.

11. Joan Borysenko, *Minding the Body, Mending the Mind* (Reading, MA: Addison-Wesley, 1987); Richard D. Carson, *Taming Your Gremlin* (New York: Harper & Row, 1983); Deepak Chopra, *Quantum Healing* (New York: Bantam, 1989); and *Perfect Health* (New York: Harmony, 1990); and *Ageless Body, Timeless Mind* (New York: Harmony, 1993); see also Norman Cousins, *Anatomy of an Illness as Perceived by the Patient* (New York: Bantam, 1981); and *The Healing Heart* (New York: Avon, 1983); Bernie S. Siegel, *Love, Medicine & Miracles* (New York: HarperCollins, 1985); and *Peace, Love & Healing* (New York: HarperCollins, 1989); Andrew Weil, *Natural Health, Natural Medicine* (Boston: Houghton Mifflin, 1990).

12. Paramahansa Yogananda, *Man's Eternal Quest* (Los Angeles: Self-Realization Fellowship, 1975); Sri Chinmoy, *Beyond Within* (Jamaica, NY: Agni Press, 1974).

13. *Unity Magazine*, Association of Unity Churches.

We are capable
of infinite possibilities
and become limited
only when we shut the door
on new ones or
when we are not aware
that there are doors we haven't seen.

Virginia Satir
—Meditations and Inspirations

64

Reiki Miracles

Whenever Reiki therapists get together they always like to share their Reiki Miracle stories. Usually it isn't very long before Reiki therapists have their own assortment of miracles. Frequently the miracles start before the training weekend is over; sometimes they even start at the introductory workshop.

The most exciting Reiki Miracles usually take place with accidents, infants and animals—accidents because the imbalance is not yet in cellular memory; infants because their growth is so fast, and animals because they are so open and accepting.

It is important to understand that we never know what Reiki will do in any one situation. We all have free will, and Reiki will never interfere with free will. There can be many circumstances that are not obvious to us on the surface that can affect the outcome. We often think, for example, that we know exactly what we want in a given situation. This is our personality speaking, however, and our soul may disagree completely. The soul usually wins out over the personality for those on a spiritual path. This is truly the highest type of "win-win" situation.

I will give a few examples in each of the areas that Reiki works: physical, mental, emotional, spiritual, Karmic, and etheric. It can also be used for the empowerment of goals and objectives. Frequently there is overlap between the areas so I will not try to separate them into categories; I leave that up to you. Many of the names are changed so you will not be able to recognize the people, but they will recognize themselves. Some of our currently active therapists are listed by their real names, with their approval.

> Realize that you cannot help a soul unless that soul really wants help and is ready to be helped.
>
> I tell you to send that soul nothing but Love and more Love.
>
> Be still and wait, but be there when that soul turns for help.
>
> Eileen Caddy
> —Footprints on the Path

Mary is an RN who broke her arm by accidentally hitting it against a medicine cart at work one day. The doctor said she needed 6-8 weeks in a cast. As a per diem nurse she had no sick leave, and no paycheck. X-rayed after 10 days for a smaller cast, the arm was completely healed and Mary went back to work, very happy to have a paycheck again in 11 days.

Deb and Jerry had been separated for eight months after a 19-year marriage because their five sons were starting to follow in Jerry's footsteps as a "rage-a-holic" and Deb could take it no longer. Deb took Reiki in October, Jerry in November, and by January they were back together again. Jerry has had no more rage attacks, and their life has been like a honeymoon for the past three years.

Kathy lost over 60 pounds without trying after getting Reiki.

Bob had major abdominal surgery and astounded his doctors with his rapid recovery. His wife had Second Degree and he got First Degree in the hospital—while still on drugs from the surgery.

Andrew was searching for "something out there" to help him be more in touch spiritually and more emotionally balanced. After Reiki he went through a cathartic period of releasing negativity. He said, "It was like someone gave me a Golden Box and it had everything I wanted to know. It had the keys to my inner self. It is the most wonderful gift I have received in this life other than life itself."

Martina described her husband as an "8-day-a-week drunk." She was amazed when after a few weeks of her treating him, his drinking pattern changed to one or two drinks a week.

Sue came to Reiki in her early 60s with advanced emphysema. She and her husband used Reiki to stop the progression of the disease within 6 months.

Ann's past seven relationships had been long term with nice men who had no commitment to her, and then they left her for someone else. She did a Second Degree technique seven months after getting Reiki to help her find "the perfect relationship." A man she was not interested in kept asking her out. She went out with him, and found out he was the perfect man for her. They have been together for over a year now, and recently became engaged and will be married later this year.

Irene was on welfare and unable to hold down a job. Within six months she was totally supporting herself with her psychic readings and classes.

Lee was in his mid 30s, had been on dialysis for several years, was yellow with jaundice and in bad health. After several months of Reiki he had learned to control the painful cramping while on the dialysis machine, felt well enough to get active in sports again, and in less than a year was able to go back to work.

Fran had Chronic Fatigue Syndrome so severely she felt unable to sit through class; not only was she able to sit through class after receiving her attunements, but her energy level increased dramatically to the point she was able to complete an educational program she had almost given up hopes of ever completing, and was able to work again.

Sue had a very large, rapidly growing breast tumor her doctor felt was cancerous. Her friend Joan gave her one hands-on and several absentee treatments. When she saw the specialist several days later, he found no tumor. She had the mammogram to show that it had been there only a few days before.

Annie wore gloves and a scarf that covered her head, neck, and part of her face when she came to class because her psoriasis was so extensive. She had been under treatment for it for over two years without a change. Within a month of taking Reiki the psoriasis was gone.

Evelyn was 78 and home-bound with Lou Gehrig's Disease when a neighbor gave her Reiki treatments. After the treatments she felt so much better she had me come over and initiate her at First Degree. Several months later, at her annual checkup, her Doctor was quite amazed that her cataracts and numerous breast tumors of long duration were totally gone, and she could speak without having to use her stomach muscles.

Andrew found after Reiki that his natural talents of sight, touch, and hearing were greatly enhanced. His ability to see more within the auric field increased appreciably, as did his sensitivity to people's emotional needs and his hearing of finer gradations of frequencies.

Mandy was an actress getting about 10 percent of the parts she auditioned for. Within a year that percentage was up to 80 percent, an unheard-of acceptance rate.

Noelle's walnut-sized ovarian cyst was very painful for months. Surgery was recommended if it lasted another month. She taped her hand to her stomach at night until waking up (about 4 hours). At her 6 week checkup it was gone. She was the third woman to use this technique successfully.

Kathy's 20-year-old schizophrenic son walked away from home with no money, no clothes, and no medicine. She had no word of him for over a year. After one month of absentee treatments he called and asked if he could come home.

Tracy's first kidney stone required three days in the hospital. This time the pain started and he couldn't urinate. At the hospital he held a crystal over the kidney, did Second Degree Reiki, and in 15 to 20 minutes, the pain was gone. Suddenly he really had to urinate and out popped the stone. They kept him for only four hours and the next day he went back to work.

Dr. Clem, D.C., used his Reiki to totally heal a detached retina; no surgery was needed.

MaryAnn had been a healer for years; after her attunements she had "X-Ray vision" and could look inside and see internal organs, bones, and dis-ease.

Cheri was on chemotherapy. Her white count was down to 2.9 on Monday morning. Without an increase there would be no chemo on Wednesday. She attended healing night, had acupuncture and got a shot of white-count medicine. By Wednesday afternoon the count was 9.7 so she got her chemo. She had never had that big a jump before.

Patti was doing work trade at the center. We suspected she was drinking on the job so a staff/family intervention was held and she was placed into treatment. This was not her first attempt at sobriety; she had been in and out of many treatment programs. When last heard from about a year later, she was still clean and sober.

Lynn had been on disability with severe emphysema for several years. After getting Reiki, the progression of the disease stopped and she wasn't hospitalized (the pattern had been many weeks each year of hospitalization). After full treatments for 30 days by Reiki friends her "barrel" chest was normal.

Pamela said she had been suicidal every day of her life since age 4 or 5. She had always been under a psychiatrist's care and on medication that helped her depression somewhat, but never really lifted it. Several times she had almost succeeded in committing suicide. Within 3 weeks of taking First Degree she was totally off her medications and her life began turning around. Several months later, after getting Second Degree, she was self-supporting in her own business.

Hanna's daughter was scheduled for abdominal surgery for endometriosis and two large ovarian cysts. Hanna took First Degree Reiki and treated her daughter; many others did absentee treatments. The surgeon found no tumor or endometriosis when they operated the following week.

Houses in the Los Angeles area are, I feel, rather expensive. There are 6 people who are now proud homeowners thanks to Reiki empowering techniques, and one even did it with no down payment.

Cari was a psychologist specializing in women with Epstein-Barr Virus and Chronic Fatigue Syndrome. She had difficulty working because of her own dis-ease, but after taking Reiki she experienced a sharp decrease in her symptoms and greatly improved physical and mental health.

Brigetta's Mom has had gall bladder problems since childhood and was severely limited in her diet. After getting a Reiki treatment she went to the bathroom and passed 2 heaping handfuls of sand, and now can eat anything.

Thomas and Fred took Reiki together. Thomas already had full-blown AIDS, but was making many changes to help his quality of life—diet, positive thought, alternative medicine, etc. When Thomas made his transition some months later Fred said the process was greatly eased because he was able to help soften Thomas's passing, keeping his hand on Thomas' heart during the transition. Fred said he did not feel helpless; and that it was one of their most beautiful moments together.

Linda was considering giving up drugs but she had no money for a treatment program. She came to a workshop, felt intuitively that Reiki was the answer for her, started her work trade, took her class and quit drugs completely.

Karry had been a quadriplegic for about 6 years and unable to dress or do much for himself. After 6 months of Second Degree he had use of both thumbs, and within a year was able to put his T-shirts on and off by himself.

Joanie was an artist and frequently went out in the desert alone to paint. After Reiki she developed the ability to communicate with Spirit. From then on she felt very safe and protected by her newfound friends.

Harry was employed as a part-time teacher in a private school at very low pay and with no benefits. Soon after using a Second Degree technique he was hired by the public schools full time with full benefits and excellent pay.

Joe had cancer for over a year, had been on chemotherapy for most of that time, and had been given 4 months to live when he met Reiki. Immediately he found he no longer had his "Saturday after Chemo" feeling, he was feeling better, had more energy and had a brighter outlook on life. About a year later he was given a clean bill of health by Sloan Kettering Cancer Center.

Jerry was in great pain from the rotator cuff in his shoulder before surgery. A friend started treating him and the pain left. After surgery the Doctors were amazed at the speed of his recovery, and that he didn't need physical therapy.

Joe had a twenty-year history of severe PTSD (post traumatic stress disorder). A year after taking Reiki he was driving through an area where he heard gunshots. In the past, he would undoubtedly have been hospitalized for weeks with an acute episode of PTSD. Now, instead of falling to the floor and hiding in terror, he calmly drove home.

Karen used empowerment techniques to get a job. Two years later she was making 42-1/2 times the income she had been making when she started the job, plus she had full fringe benefits.

Linda's arm froze, became swollen and extremely painful. Three doctors decided it was bursitis, gave her medication and said to come back in a month. She left their office at 9:30 P.M. At 10:30 P.M. she suddenly found she could move her arm, almost pain free. The next day she found out I had been doing my daily attunements/treatments at 11:30 P.M. in Colorado (that was 10:30 P.M. in L.A.), and realized that was what she had tapped into.

Laurie was extremely overweight all her life. In the first three months after taking Reiki she lost 30 pounds without trying. She decided if it was going to be this easy she would actually try. She joined Weight Watchers. The last time I saw her she had lost over 130 pounds and was within 15 pounds of her goal.

Tracy had started seeing Spirit shortly before taking Reiki. Soon after Reiki he started seeing dark spots in the etheric field indicating pain, then light fuzzy areas indicating stress. Next was energy as metal chunks, then as rods, then as energy spikes. When he physically removes these rods, he sees energy start to flow again.

Engrid liked her work and her boss. Because of company problems, her pay was cut in half and she never knew from week to week if she would get a paycheck. After she used a Reiki technique to manifest the perfect job and went on numerous interviews, she finally got an offer of a job which was good but not at the pay scale she desired. She spent 4 days unsuccessfully playing telephone tag trying to accept the job even though the pay was low. The new boss called her at 7:00 A.M. and offered her $5,000 more per year to take the job.

Anita had bowel cancer, was in great pain, had little mobility and was scheduled for surgery. On the second day of class she walked in without effort and was almost pain free. She did not look at all like the woman in class the night before. The following week she went ice skating for the first time in two years. Shortly after she got Reiki she had surgery and, unexpectedly, the tumor was found to be totally self-contained. She made no changes in her life style and I am sorry to have to report that two years later the cancer recurred and she made her transition.

Martin's 4-year-old nephew broke his collarbone and was put in a neck brace. Martin did absentee treatments daily on his nephew. After five days the Doctor re-X-rayed and found the collarbone totally healed.

Joe, a well known actor, had many wonderful feelings during his Reiki attunements. Some months after taking Reiki he was the director for a famous TV show in which one of the characters is transformed into a "Being of Light." **REIKI??**

Deb's Chihuahua had her leg broken on a Saturday night. When the vet set the leg, she said it would need surgery, but the soonest she could do it was the following Friday. Each day one of Deb's sons (all of whom have First Degree Reiki) stayed home from school and held the dog all day, and in the evenings Deb and her husband Jerry took over. On Friday the vet said no surgery was needed.

Harry was very active in high school sports. At 16 he broke his arm in a sports accident (4th time). He had First Degree and his Mom had Second. Both treated it extensively. Ten days later the cast was taken off and the arm was fully healed. All three times before, it had been in a cast for many weeks, just as the doctor had predicted.

I started wearing glasses in junior high and my eyes had gotten progressively worse over the years. After Reiki they leveled off for several years and they have gotten progressively better ever since. One year they were 1 full diopter better in each eye; this year 1/2 diopter better.

Albert found his astrology practice multiplied five-fold the week after Reiki. He says "the symbols of astrology became more alive for me—they seem to be living with meaning, not dead with 'characteristics.'" His instinct to see from the client's point of view and contribute clarity to life situations has been greatly enhanced, as has his creativity, concentration, and perception.

Noelle noticed after Second Degree that often she will know what someone is going to say before it is said, and whether the person is speaking their truth—a very helpful tool for a psychotherapist.

Mike was a successful Public Defender, who was winning more than half of his trial cases. After receiving Reiki he went on a tear—winning 11 out of his next twelve trials.

Carol was on chemotherapy and was given 90 days to live when diagnosed with cancer of the spine, bone, breast, lungs and liver in 1988. When she and her husband Bill came in on the weekend of November 17, 1990, for First & Second Degree Reiki Carol had what I call a "death mask." By January 1st she looked fine, had good color and was obviously in less pain. By February, three months later, the cancer was out of her liver, her CEA (cancer count in the blood) had shown a dramatic drop and her CA 15.3 (Cancer Tumor Marker, i.e., how big the tumor is) had dropped approximately **30 POINTS**—also considered a dramatic drop in size. As of August 1993 Carol has shown remarkable improvement, is feeling much better, and has no new lesions of the spine (many of the old ones have healed). The lung cancer is down to the size of a silver dollar and Carol is doing great.

The explanation of all your
problems, difficulties, and triumphs
in life boils down to this:
Life is a state of consciousness.
This is the beginning and the end.
This is the final step in metaphysics.
All the other steps lead to this.

Emmett Fox

Reiki Research

HEMOGLOBIN AND HEMATOCRIT

Acceptable scientific research on Reiki is limited. Most of what we have is anecdotal data. One scientifically structured piece of research was done by one of my students, Wendy Wetzel, several years ago. Wendy was working for a Masters Degree in Nursing at Sonoma State University.[1] She used the protocol developed by Dr. Dolores Krieger, professor of Nursing at New York State University, for measuring the effects of Therapeutic Touch. [2] By substituting Reiki for Therapeutic Touch as the modality of treatment, she was able to measure the effects of Reiki on human in-vivo hemoglobin and hematocrit, which are measurements of the oxygen-carrying capabilities of the blood.

To secure the data, Wendy drew blood from class volunteers on Friday evening before First Degree class started, and again on Saturday after class was finished. To be sure that location was not a factor, Wendy worked with me at classes in Berkeley, San Francisco, and San Diego; to be sure it was not just one teacher I taught some classes, Will taught some and we taught some together. The same measurements were taken on a control group which met for a non-Reiki healing class for the same length of time. In the control group there were no changes in anyone's hemoglobin or hematocrit levels in the 24-hour period. In the Reiki classes, **everyone's** hemoglobin and hematocrit levels showed **statistically significant changes** in the 24 hour period. Just as might be expected with a balancing energy, some levels went up and some went down.[3]

At the same time and with the same people, we took blood pressure measurements—a test that was most interesting, although it did not adhere to the stricter protocols necessary for measuring blood pressure. In the control group there were no changes in anyone's blood pressure range: measurements that were high in the beginning remained high, and normal remained normal. In the Reiki classes, everyone with normal blood pressure remained within normal range; everyone with high blood pressure returned to normal levels, and one woman with chronic low blood pressure had hers come up to normal. When I saw her some months later she said that for the first time in her life she had gone through a whole winter in San Francisco with warm hands and feet.

This research underlines the importance of knowing whether the people you are working on are taking any balancing medication. You must educate them to the necessity of carefully monitoring their medication needs. It is common for people taking blood pressure medications, thyroid, insulin, psychiatric medications, etc., to find a **dramatic decrease** in their medication needs. Some examples are:

- Tom's doctor was able to decrease his lithium dosage until he was completely off medication within one year of taking Reiki, after twelve years of lithium treatment. Tom learned to control both his manic and his depressive phases for himself with his Reiki;

- Teresa was down to half the thyroid medications she had been on for twenty years after two years with Reiki;

- Bonnie was able to decrease her insulin by half within a year;

- Elizabeth's father was totally off the high blood pressure medications he had been on for more than twelve years after one month of absentee treatments;

- Noelle's oral asthma medications are down to one quarter, the previous dosage of two years standing; in addition the four inhalers that she used four times a day, each are down to two inhalers morning and evening.

BIOFEEDBACK AND BLOOD PRESSURE

Another piece of scientifically designed research was done by Reiki Master Teacher, Penny Devine, as part of a research project at The Evergreen State College, in Olympia, Washington.[4] In the previous study we followed strict protocols in taking blood pressure; however we could not fully rule out other possible factors during the 24-hour period. In this study, however, Penny worked closely with professionals in both biofeedback and health, to assure the validity of the results.

Penny used measurements of vital statistics, biofeedback data and self report to secure her data (see Reiki Miracles chapter for "self report" or anecdotal data as reported by Reiki Center therapists). The purpose of this study was to document the effect of Reiki on stress release response.

Data and vital signs (blood pressure, heart rate, temperature, and respiration) were taken on Reiki students at the beginning and end of the first day of a Reiki class, at the end of the complete class, and one week following the class. Clients were tested with biofeedback before a treatment began and throughout the entire treatment. Anecdotal data was determined through use of "The Change Scale," a participant profile form, and a form for self-evaluation of experiences during the Reiki class. A control group with no exposure to Reiki had the same testing at corresponding times.

The research showed an immediate confirmation, by changes on the graphs, of the therapist's perceptions of energy fluctuations. An increase in energy flow was indicated by an increase in extremity temperature, which was followed by a leveling-off of temperature at the same time as the therapist felt a decrease in the energy flow. Biofeedback Relaxation Response readings showed that all but one of the participants met the muscle relation norm, while all but three participants met the "low relaxed norm." Twelve out of seventeen surpassed this norm, experiencing even deeper relaxation, in an average time of 14 minutes. The testing of vital signs showed a significant lowering of all four indicators (blood pressure, heart rate, temperature, and respiration) during the class session.

Penny appears to have succeeded in her purpose of documenting positive effects of both Reiki treatments and Reiki training on stress/relaxation levels—in participants of both genders and a wide variety of ages, occupations, and health conditions.

Any Reiki practitioner has numerous miraculous experiences of Reiki's effects (see Reiki Miracles chapter). Hopefully these two studies will be only the beginning of scientific research on Reiki; we who live Reiki know those studies will validate the results we have seen on a daily basis over many years.

KIRLIAN PHOTOGRAPHY

Kirlian photography is a method of photographing the electro-magnetic field or aura that surrounds any living thing. This method was developed by two Russian scientists, a husband and wife team, in the 1930s.[5] Most of this country's leading Kirlian work was conducted by Dr. Thelma Moss at U.C.L.A. Her work is still considered a classic in the field. Although I have not had access to the quality of equipment Dr. Moss used, I have had the opportunity to participate with many different Kirlian photographers for extremely interesting results. Usually we have taken photographs before and after Reiki attunements or Reiki treatments. The shift in each person's energy field has always been both dramatic and unique.

One professional Kirlian photographer told me he could almost always recognize a Reiki person because their auric field was so much larger and more uniform than the average person he photographed.

Another method of photography, "Aura Photographs," is fun to work with although not scientifically valid. Therefore it should not be considered in the same category as Kirlian Photography. You may have the opportunity to have both Kirlian and Aura photographs done at "New Age" expos and conferences and can observe your own "Before-After" effects.

DOWSING

Within esoteric methods of research, dowsing is an ancient technique of discerning energy fields. Dowsing is probably best known because of the work of "water witches" in locating water, usually in farming areas. Today dowsing is used to determine "ley lines" (an English term for energy fields within the earth), electromagnetic fields (EMFs), and pathogenic fields of energy for buildings and land. Dowsing is also used to determine the auric fields of a person (and any problems relating to it), appropriate foods, Bach Flower remedies and homeopathic remedies, vitamins, etc., and for communicating with your higher self for spiritual guidance.

Dowsing is extremely easy to learn.[6] It may take you quite some time, however, to develop a high level of confidence in your answers. There are two primary methods of dowsing that I am aware of:

RODS — these can be "L" rods, or "Y" rods

PENDULUM — this can be anything that hangs from a string or chain.

When dowsing with "L" Rods to measure the auric field both before and after Reiki treatments or attunements, we have consistently found an extensive increase in the size of the aura. As an example, on several occasions different people have dowsed my auric field while I am teaching and have found it to be between 40 and 60 feet in radius, compared to an everyday reading that is between 1 and 5 feet.

A pendulum can be used to measure the length of the beam of energy coming from the hand chakra and fingertips both before and after Reiki attunements. The change in the force of the pendulum swing has always been quite dramatic.

Hélène Bernet, one of our Master Therapists, is a university professor in Belgium. As a certified geobiologist, she has done years of extensive research on dowsing and is one of the finest authorities that I know on the subject. Unfortunately her writings are all in French and not yet available in English. When Hélène took her Reiki training, we measured the energy field coming from her fingertips after each attunement. She frequently uses this measurement to evaluate life experiences. Here, in her own words, is her experience:

REIKI EXPERIENCES OF A DOWSER....Some Reiki I and II events, as analyzed by a radiesthesist.
As an Aikido and Tai Ji Quan practitioner, I had a good etheric body (three feet and more) and plenty of energy pouring from my fingertips.
During the steps of initiation (First Degree), this energy was successively pouring from the palm only, separated between palm and fingertips, then pouring from both. My etheric body extended and finally blew up to fill the room with the initiation to the Second Degree.
More precisely:
First Degree
First attunement: stopped energy from fingertips,
Second attunement: gave the energy (full spectrum of twelve colours) to the palm,

73

Third attunement: separated the colours like a double rake, pouring half of the spectrum from the palm and half from the fingertips in alternate colours, like: even numbers from the palm and uneven numbers from the fingertips,
Fourth attunement: restored the full spectrum for both, all colours pouring as well from the palm as from the fingertips.
The size of my etheric body doubled.

Second Degree
This initiation blew up the size of my etheric body to 25 feet and more, filling the entire room so that we could not check beyond.
Soon after returning to Europe I used the Second Degree for opening the energy of a sacred place in Morvan, France.

To the best of our understanding, when no energy came out of her hands after the first attunement it appeared to be a shift of the energy into Reiki, as the energy increased dramatically from that point forward.

Hélène also has a method of measuring a person's color spectrum and found equally exciting changes in the "before-and-after" results of her attunements using this technique of measurement. Perhaps in a later edition of this book we can give you some of her results in this area.

CLAIRVOYANCE

Another esoteric tool for determining auric fields, "clear sight" or clairvoyance has been used for testing several healing modalities. More and more people are developing the ability to "see." While the ways in which people "see" often differ, the meanings are often remarkably similar. For example, symbols and colors, the energy activity and the size of the energy fields may all differ, however a uniform thread seems to run through the interpretations or meanings of what they see.[7]

Master Choa Kok Sui, developer of Pranic Healing, uses clairvoyants to check for dis-ease, blockages, etc. before a treatment and for the release of energy and changes in the dis-ease state following a treatment. Everything that is done with the Pranic technique is evaluated clairvoyantly, according to Stephen Co, the approved Pranic teacher in the United States.[8]

Rosalyn Bruyère is the founder of Southern California's well-known Healing Light Center, a center for developing one's healing talents by learning a wide variety of healing modalities. She is also author of *Wheels of Light, Vol. 1*, the first in her series of books to be published on the chakras as seen by a clairvoyant. [9]

Barbara Ann Brennan is one of the most noted teachers of energy healing modalities today. Her background is as a scientist and physicist, and she approaches the human energy field, or aura, from this perspective. Both her books[10] are filled with illustrations of clairvoyantly-seen auric fields, black and white and magnificent color plates.

Some of our talented therapists who "see" created "before and after" sketches of participants in our trainings. They recorded both visually and verbally what they saw. I have chosen some of the most interesting examples to include in the book. I hope you enjoy seeing them as much as the students , volunteers and staff did.[11]

FUTURE RESEARCH

There are numerous Reiki research projects currently being conducted around the world on a variety of subjects, and with many different modalities. I look forward to reporting the results of some of these projects in future editions of this book.

I am collecting formal anecdotal case histories of Reiki treatments. If you would like to take part in this research project, just make copies of the two page form at the end of the book, fill in the data as thoroughly as possible, and send it to the address on the form.

1. Wendy S. Wetzel, *Reiki Healing: A Physiologic Perspective and Implications for Nursing* (Sonoma, CA: Masters Thesis, Sonoma State University, 1988).
2. Dolores Kreiger, *Therapeutic Touch: How to Use Your Hands to Help or to Heal* (New York: Simon & Schuster, 1979).
3. See Appendix A, excerpts from Wetzel thesis.
4. See Appendix B, excerpts from Devine research.
5. Stanley Krippner and Daniel Rubin, eds., *The Kirlian Aura: Photographing the Galaxies of Life* (Garden City, NY: Doubleday, 1974); Ingrid S. Von Rohr, *Harmony is the Healer* (Boston: Element, 1992), pp. 110–117.
6. Joseph Baum, *The Beginner's Handbook of Dowsing* (New York: Crown, 1974); Rodney Davies, *Dowsing: The Art of Finding Hidden Things* (San Francisco: Thorsons, 1991); see also Abbé Mermet, *Principles and Practice of Radiesthesia* (Boston: Element, 1990).
7. Pamela Oslie, *Life Colors* (Novato, CA: New World Library, 1991).
8. Master Choa, *Pranic Healing* (York Beach, ME: Samuel Weiser, 1990).
9. Rosalyn Bruyère, *Wheels of Light: A Study of the Chakras, vol.I* (Sierra Madre, CA: Bon Productions, 1989).
10. Barbara Ann Brennan, *Hands of Light* (New York: Bantam, 1991); and *Light Emerging: The Journey of Personal Healing* (New York: Bantam, 1993).
11. See Appendix C, Aura sketches.

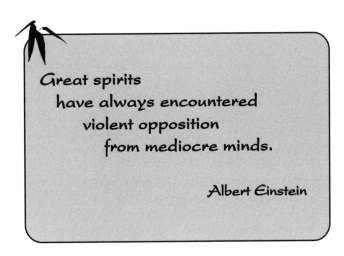

Great spirits
have always encountered
violent opposition
from mediocre minds.

Albert Einstein

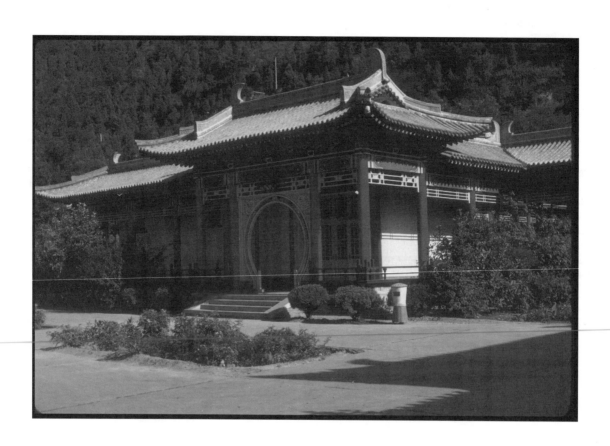

Healing Environments

I believe that we create our own worlds; we do it with our thoughts, words and actions, and usually we do it unknowingly. I like to help my students become aware of what they are creating, and help them to make changes so they can start creating what they do want in their lives rather than what they don't want.

One of the ways we create our worlds is by creating both a work and home environment. Sometimes we are not aware of the many factors which influence us: light, color, sound, etc. Vibratory energies such as these have a profound impact on both the home and work environment and assist us by enhancing healing treatments.

Creating a healing environment is an important aspect of the healing arts. Remember that with Reiki this is not a requirement—Reiki treatments or attunements can be done in the middle of a highway or a crowded room, and it still "takes." When done in a soothing, peaceful environment, however, the work is greatly facilitated. Madame Takata said that we should create a healing environment for our work.

Following is an overview of some of the things I recommend to help you create such an environment. Following this chapter you will find a bibliography of some books I have found personally useful, and that I recommend to my students to help them delve further into creating the world they desire.

> The sound of the Tinchas
> are the sound
> of the Buddha
> calling you back
> to yourself.
>
> Thich Nhat Hanh

LIGHT—One of the most harmful factors in work environments today is fluorescent lighting. Research has shown the detrimental effect of fluorescent lights: they drain energy and leave people tired, and they are agitating to most people. One way to see for yourself the effect of fluorescent lights is to have someone muscle test you both in and away from such a light (many chiropractors do this test routinely).[1]

In the 1950s Dr. John Ott[2] pioneered research about the effect of various light spectra on humans and plants; some of this work has been reconfirmed more recently by UCLA. The use of "full spectrum" fluorescent lights not only can cut down on exhaustion, it can also increase productivity and can even break through SAD, or Seasonal Affective Disorder.[3] Special light fixtures are available from a variety of sources for the treatment of SAD and possibly other situations.[4] With the original light boxes, the recommended treatment for SAD was 2 hours both morning and evening. With the newer, brighter units of 10,000 lux, only 20–30 minutes, generally in the morning, is required.

Lights can also be used to set the mood in a room. Dramatic effects can be accomplished with "up" or "down" lighting, spotlighting, etc. Color can be added for special effects by using color bulbs or color gels.[5]

COLOR—Red is different from blue, yellow from green. They are different because their energy vibrates at different frequencies. If they were the same vibration they would be the same color. That is the science of color. We are affected by these vibrations even if we are not aware of them. For example, the color red makes blood flow faster. Red cars get more tickets and are in more accidents than other colors of cars. The color "placentia pink" is used for holding tanks in many prisons across the country to calm down agitated prisoners. The color pink is usually considered a "love" energy color, while lavender and purple are considered spiritual colors, and blue and green are both considered soothing, healing colors.

Much research has been done both at universities and in industry on color and how it affects us. This is as good a place as any to begin your personal research into the ways color is affecting you. As an example: do you choose your wardrobe or the decor of your home for the way you feel or for the way you wish to feel? You will find that color is an easy and inexpensive way for you to facilitate change in your environment.[6]

COLOR CHART

COLOR	ATTRIBUTES	CHAKRA	CRYSTAL/GEM
White	Purity, Cleansing, Spiritual, Full Spectrum Elevate Energy	Above Crown	Moonstone, Opal, Diamond, Clear Quartz
Blue	Healing, Calming, Relaxation, Peace & Harmony	Throat	Sapphire, Turquoise, Aquamarine
Purple/ Indigo Royal	Healing, Psychic Knowledge, Spiritual, Universal Love	Brow	Amethyst, Lapis Sodalite
Lavender/ Violet	Nurturing of Self		Lepidolite
Pink	Love, Balance		Rose Quartz, Pink Tourmaline
Red	Vigor, Energy, Strength, Action,	Root	Ruby, Garnet
Orange	Stimulant, Sexual, Creative Reproduction	Spleen	Red Agate, Carnelian
Yellow	Joy & Happiness, Will Power, Creative, Wisdom	Solar Plexus	Tiger's eye, Citrine, Topaz
Green	Growth, Healing, Prosperity, Devotion, Good Luck	Heart	Emerald, Jade
Black	Grounding		Hematite, Apache's Tears

SOUND—The first research project I was aware of regarding sound was done by one of the midwestern agricultural universities in the 1950s. Researchers used two greenhouses, identical in all respects except that in one they played light melodious classical music, and in the other a very loud raucous rock and roll style music. The plants exposed to the light gentle music thrived and grew. The ones exposed to the loud music fell over and died. The only variable was sound—another form of vibratory energy. We are affected by the music, traffic sounds, airplane noise, loud and irritating equipment noises, etc., around us. These sounds affect us even if we have become acclimated to them and no longer consciously hear them.

The music we choose to play can help in creating a serene atmosphere for our home or business. I always use one of Will Morris's tapes, either "Helios Attunements" or "Helios Rising," when I am doing Reiki attunements or treatments. I like the energy they impart into a room.[7] Will is a musician as well as a healer (Licensed Acupuncturist and Oriental Medical Doctor), and has created music that he clinically tested before putting onto his series of tapes. Each cut was tested to be sure it helped his patients reach a healing level. Only when he had accomplished the proper healing level with the music was it placed onto the finished tape. There are other musicians whose creations I can also recommend for their healing qualities.[8] In fact I often listened to the "High Focus" tape by Brain Sync while writing this book.

PLANTS—We have known for years that plants take in carbon dioxide and give off oxygen. Now, thanks to NASA and researcher Bill Wolverton, we also know that plants can clean the air in a room, removing what might be called "typical" household pollutants: chlorine, formaldehyde, tobacco, hydrocarbons, etc. Their research showed that these "silent" pollutants can make indoor air up to five times dirtier that the air outside.[9] They also found that certain plants removed some toxins better than others and that the best all round air cleaner was the old-fashioned spider plant.

THE TOP POLLUTION FIGHTERS[10]

Plant	Percentage of pollutant removed from chamber over 24 hours
CARBON MONOXIDE	
Spider plant (Chlorophytum elatum)	96%
Golden pothos (Epipremnum aureum)	75%
BENZENE	
English ivy (Hedera helix)	90%
Peace lily (Spathiphyllum "Mauna Loa")	80%
Marginata (Dracaena marginata)	79%
FORMALDEHYDE	
Spider plant (Chlorophytum elatum)	86%
Mass cane / Corn cane (Dracaena massangeana)	70%
Golden pothos (Epipremnum aureum)	67%
TRICHLOROETHYLENE	
Potted mum (Chrysanthemum morifolium)	41%
Peace lily (Spathiphyllum "Mauna Loa")	23%
Warneckii (Dracaena deremensis "Warneckii")	20%

NASA also determined that a 10 to 12 inch plant would clean the air in a 100 square foot area. Now you can get out the measuring tape and find out what it will take to keep your air clean.

NEGATIVE IONS—We all know how delightful it feels to be down by the ocean, by a babbling brook, or in the forest. What you may not be aware of is that you feel so good in these areas, to a large extent, because of the presence of negative ions.

An overabundance of positive ions is carried by the winds coming off the deserts, such as the Santa Ana winds or the Siroccos, and these winds all have a reputation of making people behave irrationally. Many people believe that suicide, murder, assault, and accident behaviors increase during periods of high concentrations of positive ions.

To be balanced, our auric fields should have an equal amount of negative and positive ions. If we are going to have either in excess, it is best for it to be the negative ones. You can create those same sensations in your home with candles, waterfalls, negative ion generators, or by taking showers (running water generates negative ions).

CRYSTALS— Many people consider working with crystals to be a very "New Age" phenomenon, when actually the knowledge of using crystals was written about in the Bible. Placement of gemstones (crystals) on the priest's robe for power and healing, and the amethyst stone for "those who imbibe too much," are both in the Old Testament of the Bible.[11]

Each crystal gives off its own energy based on its color, hardness, clarity, cut, size, etc. By having crystals in your home and office environment, you are making a conscious choice to bring in specific energies to affect the energies of the space. (A crystal can even"pass" as a paperweight in the most traditional of offices.) Wearing gemstones, in the form of jewelry, has long been an acceptable enhancement of one's presence and brings the energy of the stone into one's auric field. Some people incorporate crystals into their healing treatments, whether with Reiki, massage, or other holistic modalities.

The number of wonderful books available today is almost endless, but I will list a few I have found enjoyable. If you choose to go deeper into the study of crystals I suggest taking a seminar with one of the many noted teachers around the country.[12]

DIAGNOSING AND CURING OUR PERSONAL ENVIRONMENT

Environmental Pollutants/S.O.S. (Sick Office Syndrome) — More and more we are hearing about homes and office buildings in which no one can live or work without getting ill. Recently I read of two government buildings in Florida which had to be closed and which will cost millions of dollars to make habitable. Last year in Sacramento officials had to evacuate a state office building and take many of the occupants to a local hospital for treatment because the building was making them ill. The same thing happened a few years ago in San Diego. What are the causes?[13] There are several that I am aware of:

- Airtight buildings that recirculate air filled with those "typical" household pollutants we spoke of earlier as well as viruses, germs, etc.
- Building construction that uses materials (carpet, paint, paneling, fabrics, glue, wallboard, etc.) that "out-gas" such things as formaldehyde for extended periods of time.
- Construction that does not take into consideration the local conditions of heat, humidity, sunshine, rain, etc.

ELECTROMAGNETIC FIELDS (EMFs)—EMFs are the "hot" topic of the 90s. Newspapers across the country and national magazines are reporting the latest findings regarding high power lines and transformers, and their effect on the environment. Within the home/work environment, we have such things as dimmer switches, electric blankets, computers, TVs, electric razors, hair dryers, microwave ovens, cellular phones, fluorescent lights, and radar guns. The more "hi-tech" our homes and offices become, the more we create environments that are toxic to the physical and mental health of a growing number of people.

One way to lessen the effects of EMFs in your home and office is to cut down on the number of electric appliances you use. However, this is not an acceptable solution for many people who want more, not less, hi-tech equipment. For those who are unwilling to give up the electrical lifestyles (and that's most of us), there are both hi-tech and esoteric tools for neutralizing these fields of energy. Learning to identify and neutralize these fields is a fascinating art that you may find interesting.[14]

FENG SHUI— also called The Chinese Art of Placement, deals with the Chi, or energy, of land, rooms or buildings just as Reiki deals with the Chi, or energy, of a person. When a person's energy is stagnant, they have dis-ease; if there is stagnant energy in a building or in land there are blockages in the lives of those who live there. The blockages will relate to the areas of their lives where the Chi is stagnant. Feng Shui is an ancient art, roughly 3,000 years old, that was developed at about the same time as the I Ching. In the Orient many people will not buy, rent, or build unless the land and house pass a Feng Shui inspection first. The Feng Shui master, or the beginning Feng Shui student, first diagnoses the problems, then corrects them with a variety of "cures." This method of diagnosing and curing is equally effective for home and business, and for land, buildings, and rooms.

Many aspects of Feng Shui are extremely complex; however, the tools for diagnosing and curing are easy to use, and the basics can be learned in a short class or from books listed in the bibliography.[15]

> If you have built castles
>   in the air,
>   your work need not be lost,
>   that is where they should be.
>
> Now put the foundations
>   under them.
>
>   Henry David Thoreau

On a personal note: when I was introduced to this art several years ago, I loved the way it fit into my past training as an Interior Designer (that was in my life before both counseling and Reiki). Teaching Feng Shui gives me the opportunity to expand the balancing of Chi for my students—from their bodies to their homes and offices. Most people who are drawn to one form of energy work seem to be naturally drawn to other energy balancing modalities. As you grow in your Reiki, you, too, will discover additional forms of energy work that appeal to you. I'm sure you will enjoy the search.

When you consider the total person—the mind, body and soul, as well as both the work and home environment—then you can bring balance to all these areas.

>   **Then,**
>
>   **and only then,**
>
>   **will total HEALING**
>
>   **take place.**

1. John Diamond, *Your Body Doesn't Lie* (New York: Warner, 1989).
2. John N. Ott, *Health and Light* (Old Greenwich, CT: Devin-Adair Co., 1973); and *Light, Radiation & You: How to Stay Healthy* (Old Greenwich, CT: Devin-Adair Co., 1985).
3. American Psychiatric Association, *Diagnostic and Statistical Manual of Mental Disorders,* Third Edition, Revised DSM-III-R (Washington, DC: American Psychiatric Association, 1987), pp. 218-224; and Angela Smyth, *Seasonal Affective Disorder* (London: Thorsons, 1990).
4. Environmental Lighting Concepts, Inc. (Ott-Light Technology) 1214 West Cass St., Tampa, FL 33606 (800) 842-8848. Fax: 813-626-8790, Website: www.ott-lite.com.
5. Joseph Lieberman, *Light: The Medicine of the Future* (Santa Fe, NM: Bear & Co., 1991).
6. Linda Clark, *The Ancient Art of Color Therapy* (Old Greenwich, CT: Devin-Adair Co., 1975); Reuben Amber, *Color Therapy* (Santa Fe, NM: Aurora Press, 1983); Edwin Babbitt, *The Principles of Light & Color,* Faber Birren, ed. (Secaucus, NJ: Citadel Press, 1967).
7. Audio tapes by William Morris, "Helios Rising" (Santa Monica, CA: Helios, 1984); and "Helios Attunements" (1988).
8. Steven Halpern, "Spectrum Suite" (San Anselmo, CA: Inner Peace Music); and Kelly Howell, "Brain Sync" series (Santa Fe, NM: Brain Sync Corp.).
9. Peter Callahan, "A Healthy Room is a Leafy Room," *Omni Magazine*, Sept. 1993, p. 28.
10. "Cleaning Your Indoor Air: Mum's the Word," *New Age Journal,* pp. 20–22.
11. See Appendix D.
12. Uma Silbey, *The Complete Crystal Guidebook* (San Francisco: U-Read Publications, 1987); Katrina Raphaell, *Crystal Enlightenment* (Santa Fe, NM: Aurora Press, 1985); and *Crystal Healing* (Santa Fe, NM: Aurora Press,1987); see also Dael Walker, *The Crystal Healing Handbook* (Pacheco, CA: Crystal Co., 1988).
13. Debra Lynn Dadd, *The Nontoxic Home*; and *Nontoxic, Natural, and Earthwise*; and *The Nontoxic Home & Office* (Los Angeles: J. P. Tarcher, 1986, 1990, 1992).
14. Robert O. Becker and Gary Selden, *The Body Electric* (New York: Quill Press, 1985); and Paul Brodeur, *Currents of Death* (New York: Simon & Schuster, 1989); *The Great Power-Line Coverup* (New York: Little, Brown, 1993); see also Ellen Sugerman, *Warning: The Electricity Around You May Be Hazardous to Your Health* (New York: Simon & Schuster, 1992).
15. Susan Hornik, "How to Get that Extra Edge on Health and Wealth," *Smithsonian* (August, 1993), pp. 70–75; Sarah Rossbach, *Feng Shui: The Chinese Art of Placement* (New York: Arkana, 1991); and *Interior Design with Feng Shui* (New York: Arkana, 1991).

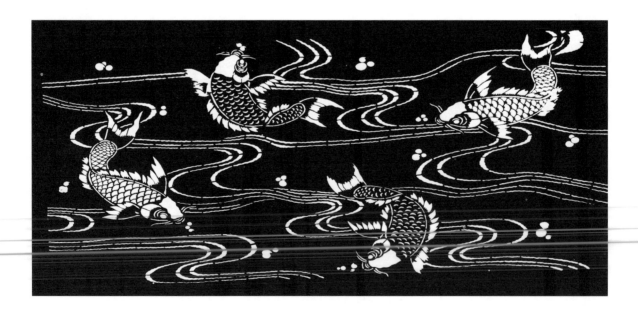

Hand Positions

My primary reason for creating a new workbook is to make sure that all the hand positions we teach are "legal." The laws in the Orient tend to be very different from those here regarding such issues as touching another individual. Many of the original hand positions taught for treating another person with Reiki are illegal in any part of the United States. Using the new hand positions shown in this manual will give you the same results as the classical positions, while remaining legally and ethically appropriate.

The second reason is my desire to incorporate into a more comprehensive manual the vast new levels of knowledge we have gained over the last 15 years regarding how Reiki works. This manual is for the layperson as well as both beginning and advanced Reiki practitioners. (Remember, however, that merely duplicating the hand positions will not give you Reiki or its results; only the Reiki attunements will do that.) The knowledge shared in this section is a compilation of what I was taught about the use of Reiki, input from my students (many of them medical professionals), and my own knowledge gleaned over the years.

For each of the hand positions of a classical treatment I have provided as much information as possible regarding the way Reiki works to enhance physical, mental, emotional, and spiritual balancing, as well as its impact on the chakra system.

For the ideal classical treatment you would start in Head Position #1 and go straight through to Back Position #6, spending about 5 minutes in each position. In all hand positions, the fingers are kept gently together, and, whenever posssible, touching at the midline of the body. The chapter on "Specific Treatments" discusses special treatment protocols for problem areas.

The classical treatment takes about an hour to an hour-and-a-half. Realistically, many treatments are done on the run with far less time than this to complete them, so there are several ways you can work with Reiki: you can do a full treatment, or a short treatment, or treat where it hurts, or put your hand somewhere trusting the Reiki to know where to go. Remember, you can never do too much or too little Reiki.

Have fun and enjoy your Reiki.

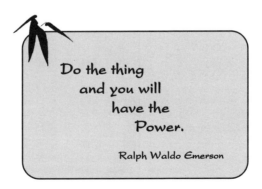

Do the thing and you will have the Power.

Ralph Waldo Emerson

Will Morris, O.M.D. has contributed the "Oriental Medicine" information for each position to give you added insights into the workings of Reiki and the tradition from which it came.

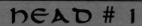

HEAD # 1

CHAIR TREATMENT
- OTHER ➤

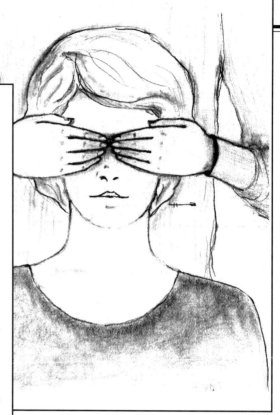

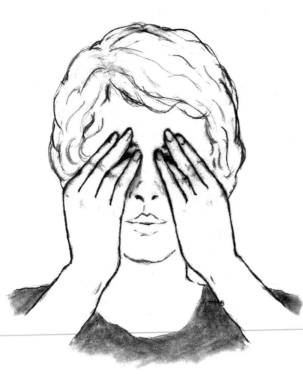

SELF TREATMENT ▲

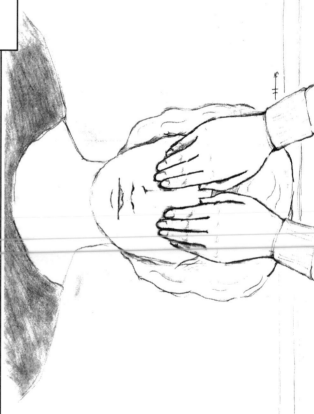

TABLE TREATMENT
- OTHER ➤

Placement of Hands

Both hands are placed gently over the eyes.

Physical

Eyes and any condition relating to eyes—nearsightedness, farsightedness, glaucoma, cataracts, detached retina, etc.;
Sinuses, colds and flu;
Pineal and pituitary glands;
Teeth;
Jaws—TMJ (temporomandibular joint dysfunctions);
Headaches.

Mental & Emotional

Clarity in one's life;
Ability to see what is needed—relationships, career, changes, etc.;
Relaxation and stress reduction.

Spiritual

Help to get centered—to go within;
Meditation;
Activation of internal light (i.e., flashes of light, kaleidoscopes of color, pictures of past lives or current events).

Chakra

Third Eye;
Insight, ability to "see" on other levels;
Used for psychic and spiritual development.

Oriental Medicine

The third eye, one's vision of the world and the ability to face it. Clarity of vision unfolds with treatment of this area; vision to realize one's destiny, where one is headed. Treatment of this area enhances clairvoyance which is clear seeing. Sinus cavity congestion can act as a block to a world connection through the senses involved with this position. Sight, taste, and scent are deeply influenced through the healing power of Reiki administered here.

Notes

_____

_____

_____

_____

_____

HEAD # 2

CHAIR TREATMENT
- OTHER ➤

SELF TREATMENT ▲

TABLE TREATMENT
- OTHER ➤

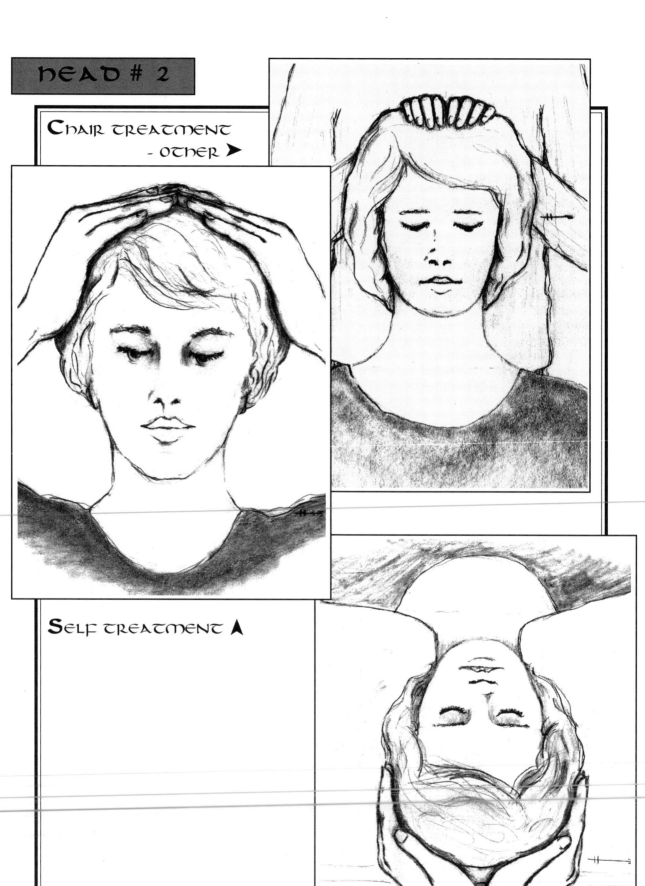

Placement of Hands

Both hands are placed on the top of the head with fingers or side of hands touching.

Physical

Balances right/left brain activity;
Inner ear infections—equilibrium problems, motion sickness (inner ear, vertigo);
Eye stem problems;
Seizures;
Pineal, pituitary;
Hypothalamus, limbic system of brain;
Headaches;
Endorphin/pain release;
Shock.

Mental/Emotional

Balancing mental/emotional problems;
Depression, anxiety, manic-depressive mood swings, creativity;
Right/left hemisphere balance;
Studying and retention of knowledge;
Memory;
Calmness;
Creativity.

Spiritual

Tap into higher consciousness;
"Cowlick is umbilical cord to Universe."

Chakra

Crown chakra.

Oriental Medicine

The crown center lends direct knowledge. This is the ability to know right action without undue mental effort. The balancing of the right and left brain take place here. It is a place of divine inspiration. The universal healing power of Reiki transmits to the whole organism through the vascular, neurological and energetic conduits finding their meeting place here; here within the thousand petaled lotus.

Notes

_____

_____

_____

_____

_____

HEAD # 3

CHAIR TREATMENT
- OTHER ➤

SELF TREATMENT ▲

TABLE TREATMENT
- OTHER ➤

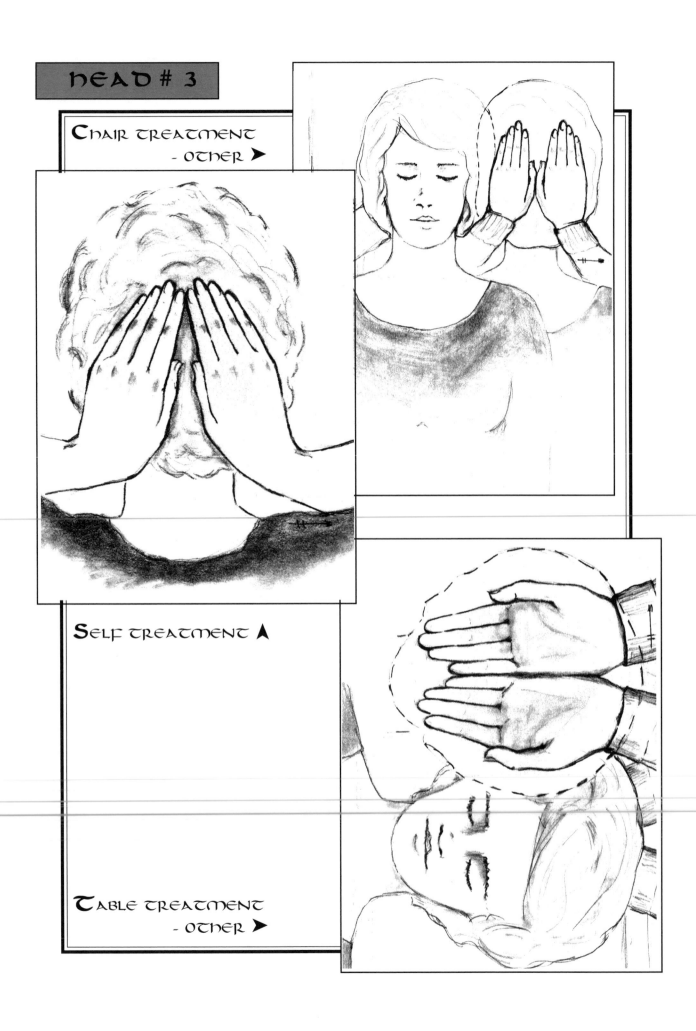

Placement of Hands

Both hands placed up the center back of the head, touching, with fingertips or lower palm of hands on base of skull.

Physical

Treats old brain/reptilian brain;
Governs basic bodily functions, tells heart to beat, lungs to breathe, food to digest, etc.;
Asthma, emphysema, pneumonia, various heart/circulatory problems, sleep disorders;
Treats back of eye stem;
More left/right hemisphere balancing;
More inner ear.

Mental/Emotional

Past life and past dream recall;
Very nurturing position for self/others by "cradling the head" relaxation;
Pituitary and pineal (balancing of the glands).

Spiritual

Some people consider that Spirit enters and leaves at this area of the head;
Secondary position for Third Eye treatment.

Oriental Medicine

Found around the lower brain stem, this area addresses unconscious urges and patterns. Use this area to treat addictive behavioral patterns. This area is stimulated by the Rosicrucians to generate a state of wakefulness and mindfulness. Certain esoteric schools consider the lower brain stem to be an essential link to the greater beingness.

Notes

CHAIR TREATMENT
- OTHER ➤

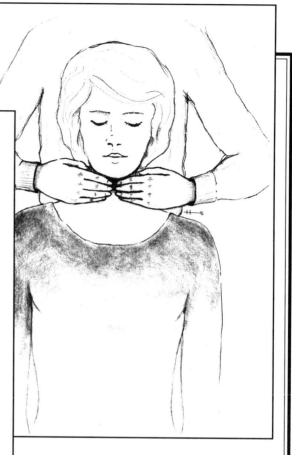

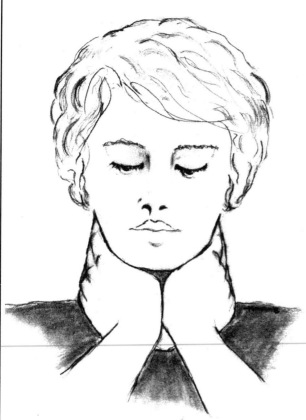

SELF TREATMENT ▲

TABLE TREATMENT
- OTHER ➤

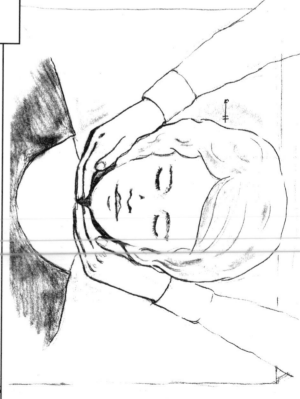

Placement of Hands

Both hands are gently placed on the throat with fingertips, or base of palms, touching over the thyroid.

Physical

Thyroid, for balancing metabolism (high or low);
Parathyroids for calcium/magnesium assimilation—especially important for women before, during, and after menopause;
Osteoporosis;
Carotid artery for treating blood, especially blood entering the brain;
Balances high or low blood pressure;
Hemoglobin/hematocrit;
Circulation;
Strokes;
Probably effective in assisting medications which cross blood/brain barrier;
Might affect balancing medications;
Sore throat, tonsillitis, larynx;
Lymphatic drainage.

Mental/Emotional

Major power center for the body; control by tone of voice and words we speak, codependency recovery because of power/control issues;
Especially important for anger and rage;
Self-confidence, anxiety, stage fright—particularly pertinent for performers;
Stabilizing;
Communication.

Chakra

Throat.

Oriental Medicine

This is the throat chakra. It is evident with the revelation of truth. Responsibility is the key word which reflects the ability to respond. Every acupuncture meridian traverses this area; comfort here is essential to optimal well-being.

Notes

_____

_____

_____

_____

_____

_____

_____

FRONT # 1

CHAIR TREATMENT
- OTHER ▶

SELF TREATMENT ▲

TABLE TREATMENT
- OTHER ▶

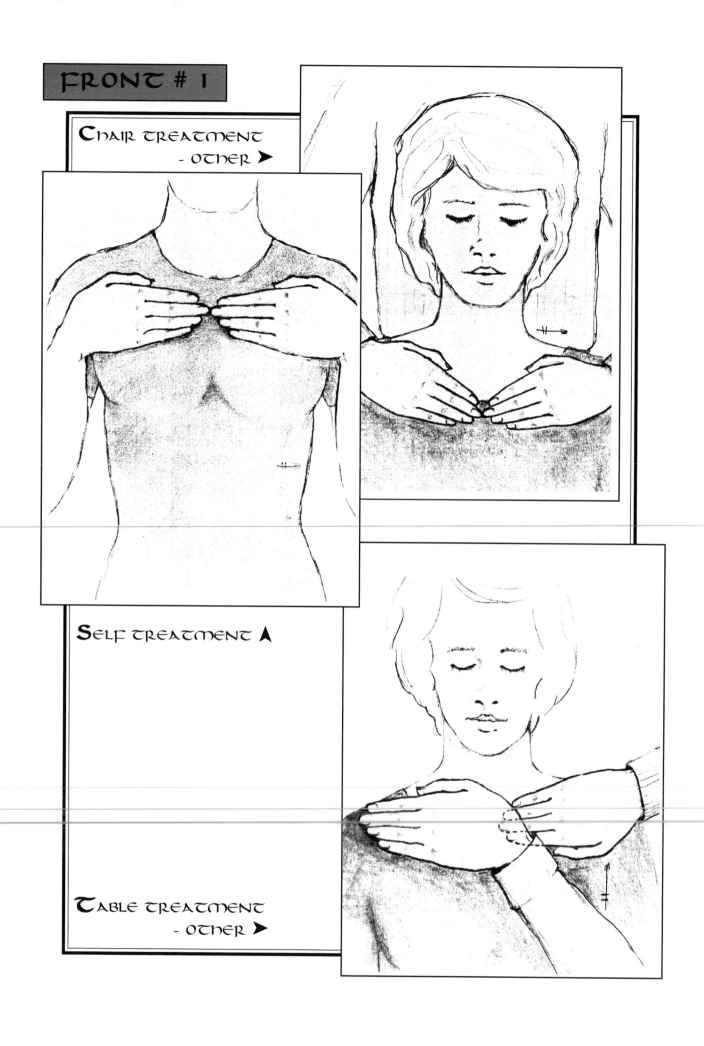

Placement of Hands

Place both hands on the upper chest over the thymus with the fingers touching.

Physical

Thymus—immune system/immune system disorders and autoimmune disorders such as lupus, arthritis, chronic fatigue, Epstein-Barr Virus, HIV+, AIDS, cancer;
Lymphatic drainage;
Lungs—asthma, emphysema, pneumonia, lung cancer;
Physical heart and any heart problems, circulation.

Mental/Emotional

Emotional heart problems—broken heart, grief, joy, happiness/unhappiness;
Balancing any strong feelings;
Entering, returning to self;
Going within;
Comforting.

Spiritual

May be the location that the spirit leaves the body at the moment of transition (death);
Unconditional love;
Compassion.

Chakra

Heart.

Oriental Medicine

Treats the heart. The heart is the throne of the spirit. When the heart is in balance, the mind is clear and memory functions well. The thymus gland is responsible for aspects of immune function. This is the determination of self and not-self. This is an important position for those who tend to lose themselves within a relationship.

Notes

FRONT # 2

CHAIR TREATMENT
- OTHER ▶

SELF TREATMENT ▲

TABLE TREATMENT
- OTHER ▶

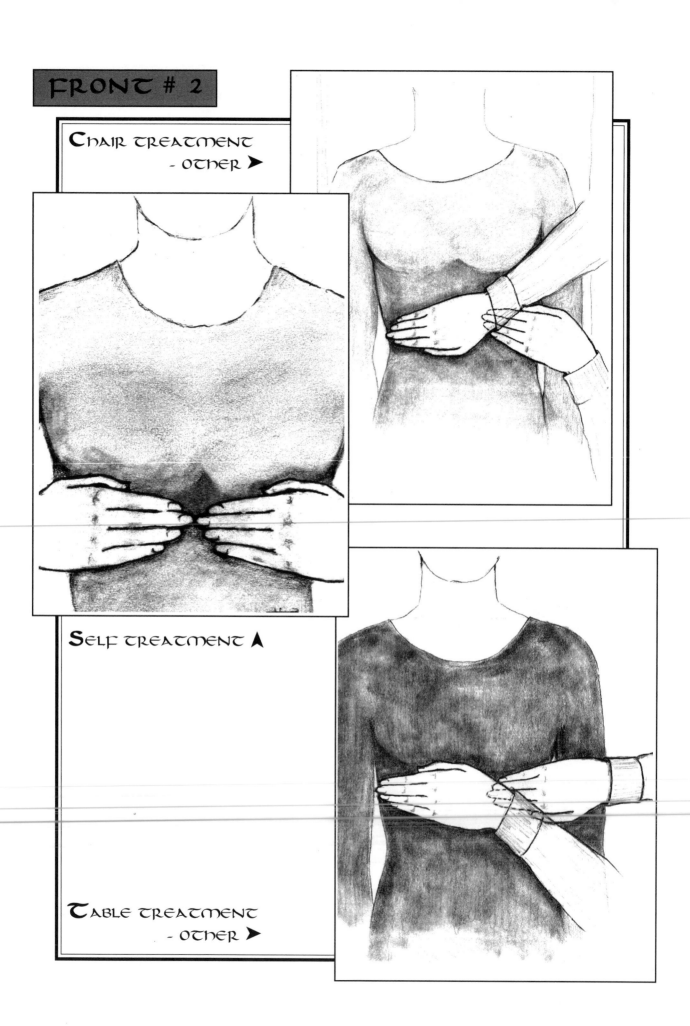

FRONT #2 & #3 (Together)

Starting from the right side to the left side, Front #2 and #3 treat the following organs, glands, etc.

Placement of Hands

Front #2—both hands are placed under the breasts, over the rib cage, with fingertips touching at the base of the breastbone.

Front #3 —both hands are placed at the waist, above it, with the fingertips touching.

LIVER
(far right side)

Physical

Primary organ for detox—not just items we usually think of, such as alcohol, which is processed in the liver, but any other toxin as well, such as the wax on the apples from the store, the pesticides/insecticides that our food has been treated with, the chemicals in the air we breathe and the water we drink—in other words, any toxic substance taken into the body in any manner that must be detoxed.

Hormonal imbalances such as PMS in women and midlife crisis in men;
Estrogen metabolized in liver;
Processes medications;
Headaches;
Metabolizes lactic acid;
Environmental allergies;
Jaundice;
Cholesterol.

Mental/Emotional

Emotionally, liver is unresolved anger issues;
Processing "sludge"—old issues/feelings.

Notes

_____

_____

GALL BLADDER
(tucked into the liver)

Physical

Produces gall/bile;
Gallstones;
Part of digestive process.

FRONT # 3

CHAIR TREATMENT
- OTHER ►

SELF TREATMENT ▲

TABLE TREATMENT
- OTHER ►

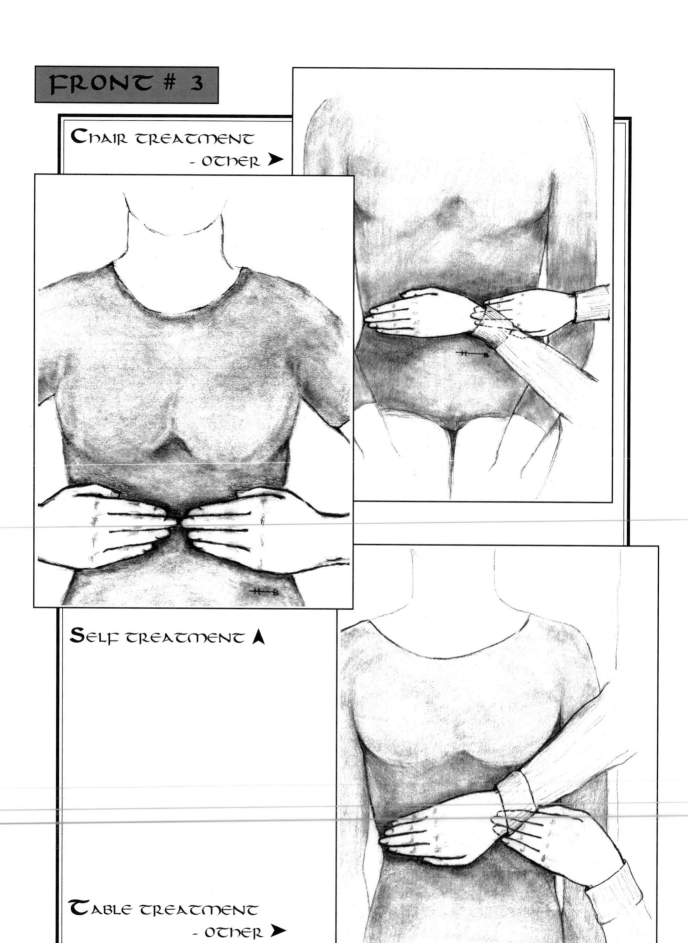

Mental/Emotional

Covers that special type of anger: "that really galled me"—the kind of anger that has bitterness to it;
Decision-making organ.

Notes

PANCREAS
(almost directly in the middle)

Physical

Handles insulin production for the body, diabetes, and hypoglycemia;
Position to treat for a quick picker-upper, when energy is low;
Control or manipulation issues;
Fear.

Mental/Emotional

For people who have too little or too much "sweetness" in their lives;
Fear;
Centering;
Increased self-esteem;
Major inner-strength center for the body (and the self).

Chakra

Solar plexus.

Notes

STOMACH
(far left side)

Physical

Digests food.

Mental/Emotional

Digests ideas.
Starts process of breaking things down into component parts.

Notes

Thoughts are things,
    they have tremendous power.

Thoughts of doubt and fear
    are pathways to failure.

When you conquer negative attitudes
    of doubt and fear you conquer failure.

Thoughts crystallize into habit
    and habit solidifies into circumstances.

Brian Adams

Neither body nor mind
must be master over us.
We must remember
that the body belongs to us
and not we to the body.

Vivekananda

SPLEEN
(behind the stomach)

Physical

Blood purifier—treat here for any infections anywhere in the body;
Manufactures T-cells and is vitally important for treatment of any immune system disorders;
Also important for autoimmune disorders such as: chronic fatigue, Epstein-Barr Virus, HIV+, AIDS, lupus, rheumatoid arthritis.

Mental/Emotional

Handles that special release of anger referred to as "venting your spleen."

Chakra

Spleen.

Oriental Medicine

Treats the solar plexus; the seat of power; organs we find here are the liver, spleen, gallbladder, and pancreas.

In Chinese medicine, the liver is considered to be the "General." Through it one has the vision to guide the forces forward in life. The emotion associated with the liver and gallbladder is anger. When naturally expressed, it is an assertive life force growing and bursting forth with the vitality of spring. Anger evolves when the expression is suppressed or thwarted due to internal or external causes.

The gallbladder is the helmsman of the ship. It is involved in the smaller daily decisions we make.

The pancreas is associated with equanimity of mind. When we ruminate or worry too much, this affects the pancreas' ability to secrete enzymes necessary to digest foods. Hence, the wisdom of quiet time and prayer before meals.

The spleen is a large lymph node which filters blood and lymph. This position is one of the most important for daily physical well-being; there are many organs here, including the diaphragm.

Notes

_____

_____

_____

_____

_____

_____

_____

_____

_____

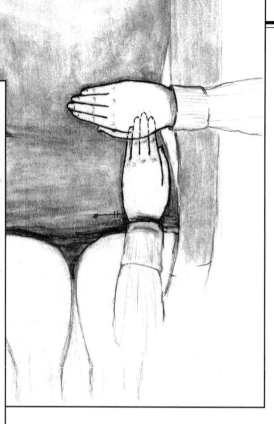

FRONT # 4 & 5

CHAIR TREATMENT LEFT SIDE OTHER ➤

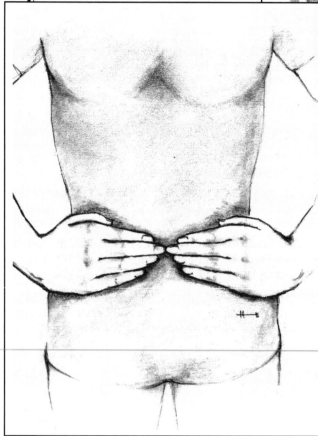

SELF TREATMENT ▲

CHAIR TREATMENT RIGHT SIDE OTHER ➤

Placement of Hands

For self treatment :
#4: place both hands at the waist, below it, with fingertips touching;
#5: place both hands so the fingertips touch on the pubic bone.

For treating another person combine the two positions:
Place one hand at the waist, below it, and the other along the hip bone;
Repeat on the other side of the body.

	Physical	Mental/Emotional
TOGETHER, THESE TREAT:	Lymphatic drainage Circulation Constipation and diarrhea Mucous conditions Flu	Emotional releases Creativity Emotional withholding Emotional "dumping"

FRONT #4

SMALL INTESTINE

Physical

Assimilates nutrients for the body.

Mental/Emotional

Assimilates ideas.

Notes

_____

_____

LARGE INTESTINE & COLON

Physical

Eliminates: waste products from body;
toxins the body is discharging.

Mental/Emotional

Eliminates people, places, things that are no longer needed in one's life (a good place to treat if you're changing, moving, breaking up a relationship, cleaning out closets, etc.).

Chakra

Sexual.

FRONT # 4 & 5

TABLE TREATMENT LEFT SIDE OTHER ➤

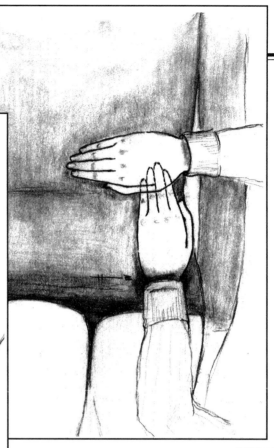

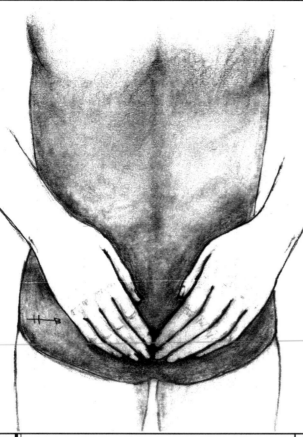

SELF TREATMENT ▲

TABLE TREATMENT RIGHT SIDE OTHER ➤

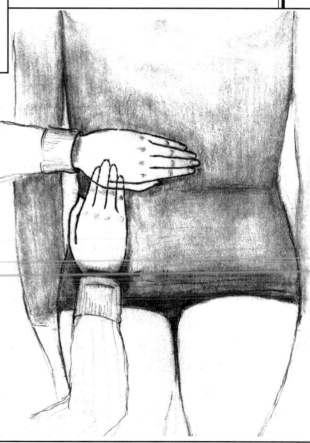

Oriental Medicine

This involves the small and large intestines. The small intestine functions to decide which nutrients we will take into our body and which ones will be left out. This also applies to other levels such as processing incoming information, emotions, and experiences.

The small intestine's metaphor is sifting and processing. When there is data overload or food overload, it is easy for stagnation to take place in the small intestine.

The large intestine involves the capacity to let go of what we don't need. When free exchange of issues and things in our life is too fast, diarrhea can result. When there is congestion in the process of letting go, constipation can be the result.

This is the second chakra; its key word is intimacy. This reflects the capacity for timely disclosure. The appropriate revelation of our story with another human being. It is also the capacity to be open and vulnerable appropriately in a relationship. This position treats sexuality as an expression of closeness and intimacy.

Notes

FRONT #5

Physical

Both male and female reproductive systems and any physical or emotional problems relating to them;
Migraine headaches (which may relate to sexual repression);
Bladder and its conditions (cystitis, etc.).

Mental/Emotional

Additional release (bladder).

Spiritual

Grounding.

Chakra

Root.

Oriental Medicine

This treats the urogenital tract and lower intestines. It is the root chakra. The root chakra key word is survival. It goes out of balance when we engage in making a living that is not aligned with our destiny. This chakra revolves around the question of right livelihood. This livelihood should contribute to the survival of Gaia, Mother Earth, as well as order, to sustain true balance in this chakra.

Notes

BACK # 1

CHAIR TREATMENT
- OTHER ▶

SELF TREATMENT ▲

TABLE TREATMENT
- OTHER ▶

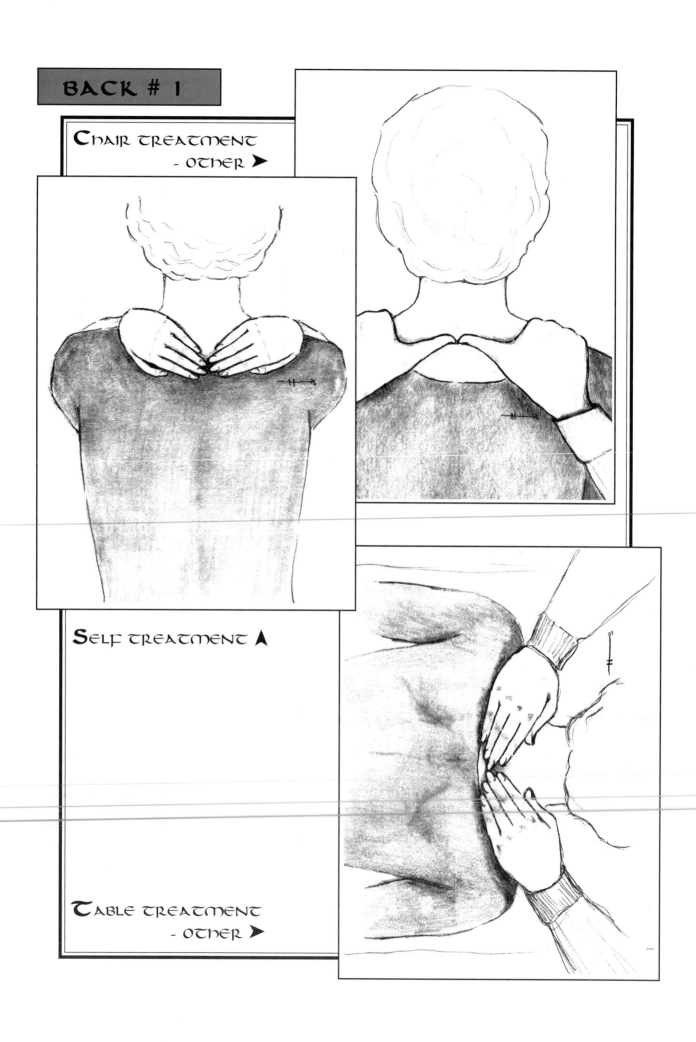

FOR ALL BACK POSITIONS

Metaphysically, difficulties of the spine indicate a lack of support, either emotional or financial, either at home or at work. All back hand positions therefore assist with this condition.

BACK #1

Placement of Hands

Drape hands over the shoulders with fingertips touching on the spine.

Physical

Starts flow of energy up/down spine;
Treats plexus of nerves that radiate around the heart/lung areas;
Treats spot on top of shoulders (the "bra-strap" spot) that is a major endorphin-releasing spot for the body. Endorphins are a natural morphine the body produces. Morphine kills pain; therefore use this position for pain anywhere in the body;
This same spot on top of shoulders is considered "gateway to the lungs" in Oriental medicine and is therefore used to treat any lung-related problem;
Flexibility.

Mental/Emotional

Flexibility;
Nape of neck is area where many people hold stress; therefore this is an excellent position to treat for stress reduction.

Oriental Medicine

This treats the throat chakra. It also stimulates and harmonizes the parasympathetic (feed or breed) nervous system. This aspect is used for people who are high-strung, nervous and tense. It stimulates the mood of a candle-light dinner or a hot bath. This position is excellent when combined with abdominal hand positions to improve digestive function through autonomic nervous system regulation.

Notes

BACK #. 2

CHAIR TREATMENT
- OTHER ►

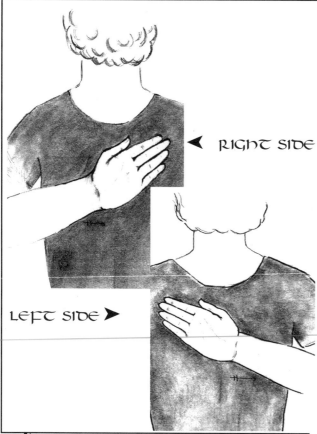

◄ RIGHT SIDE

LEFT SIDE ►

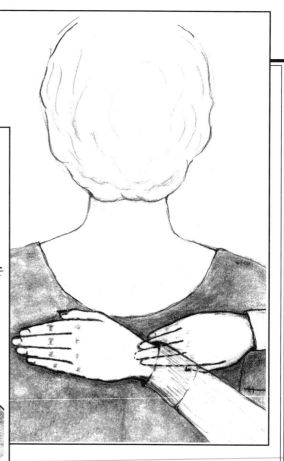

SELF TREATMENT ▲

TABLE TREATMENT
- OTHER ►

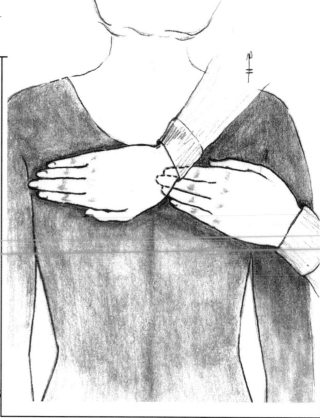

Placement of Hands

Place hands across the shoulder blades with hands touching on the spine.

Physical

Back of heart, back of lungs, and more of the spine.

Mental/Emotional

Open up to love—softening of rigidity as far as love is concerned.

Spiritual

Treat here for opening up to universal love.

Chakra

Back of heart chakra (see Front #1).

Oriental Medicine

This addresses the heart. A chakra may be closed and tight in the front or in the back. It is important to treat both sides. This spinal area is the sympathetic aspect; it can be used with the rest of the back to regulate the fight-or-flight response. This position also has acupuncture points which are used for chronic tenacious problems. This position should be used for any pattern of imbalance more than two months old.

Notes

CHAIR TREATMENT
- OTHER ➤

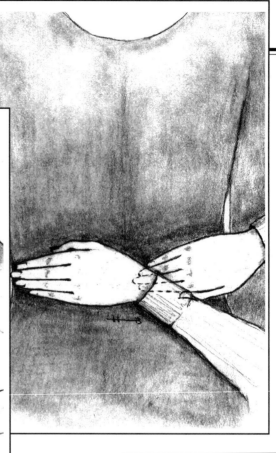

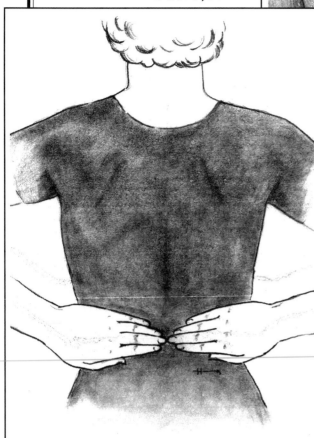

SELF TREATMENT ▲

TABLE TREATMENT
- OTHER ➤

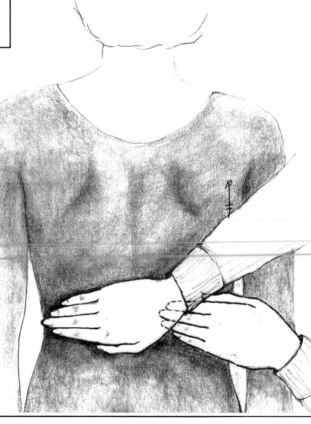

Placement of Hands

Place both hands at the waist, above it, with hands touching.

Physical

Kidneys, which filter waste products of body;
Kidney stones.

Mental/Emotional

Filter ideas and concepts that are no longer useful;
The kind of anger you feel when you are "pissed off."

Chakra

Back of the Solar Plexus (see Front #2 & #3).

Oriental Medicine

This addresses sympathetic nerve balance and digestive function as governed by the stomach, pancreas, liver, and gallbladder. It also adjusts function of the spleen. Treatment of diaphragm spasm should include this position as a focus.

Notes

BACK # 4

CHAIR TREATMENT
- OTHER ▶

SELF TREATMENT ▲

TABLE TREATMENT
- OTHER ▶

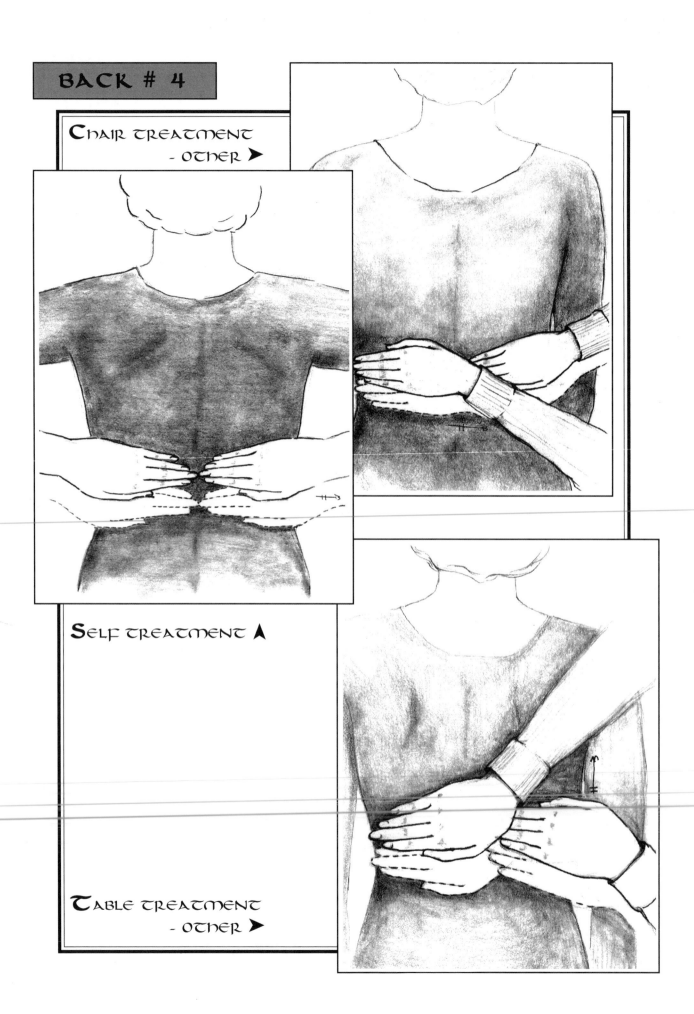

Placement of Hands

Move hands up 1/2 hand above Back #3 to cover the adrenals.

Adrenals in General

There really are no saber-toothed tigers on the freeway but your body responds as if there are. Whenever we get excited the adrenal glands pump adrenalin throughout body and then we have situations of either adrenalin overload, where the body has more adrenalin than it needs on a regular basis, or adrenal failure, where it is used too much and breaks down.

Today we must also deal with adrenal addiction, where people become addicted to the adrenalin rush. As an example, look at the movies currently produced that appeal to this addiction in both young people and adults.

Physical

Essential for immune system disorder—E-BV, CFS, HIV+, AIDS, environmental allergies, cancer, etc.;
In Oriental medicine, this is the gate of life, and should be treated for those desiring pregnancies;
It is also considered the gland of longevity, so treat here for reversing the aging trend;
More of the spine;
Back pain.

Mental/Emotional

"Fight-or-flight" mechanism and its emotional implications.

Chakra

Back of solar plexus (see Front #2 & #3).

Oriental Medicine

This primarily treats the kidneys. The Chinese consider this area to contain the gate of life. This is where the essential spark of our genetic potential is lit at conception. As the embryo develops it unfolds from this area. As such, this area relates to one's destiny. This position balances willfulness. Destiny is attained when one aligns the personal will with the will of heaven. This is fulfillment of genetic potential, or empowerment of the essence of one's being.

Notes

_____

_____

_____

_____

_____

_____

CHAIR TREATMENT
- OTHER ➤

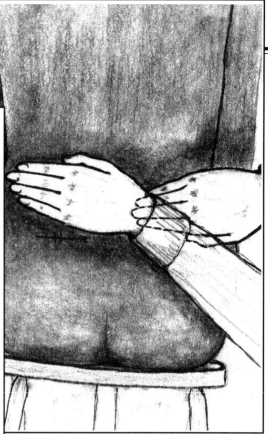

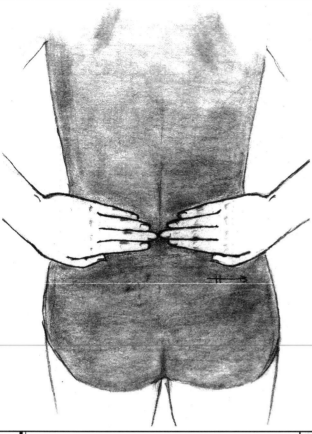

SELF TREATMENT ▲

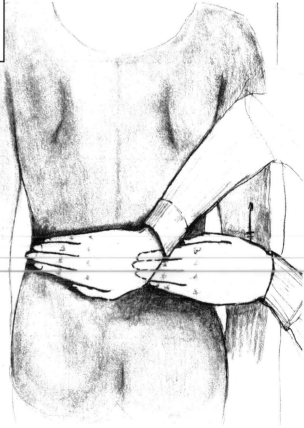

TABLE TREATMENT
- OTHER ➤

Placement of Hands

For #5 place both hands at the waist, below it, with hands touching;
For #6 place both hands across the hips with hands touching on the tailbone.

BOTH TOGETHER TREAT:

Physical	Chakra
Back of small and large intestines	Root
Back of colon	Sexual
More of spine	Spleen
Sciatic nerve problems	
Lower back pain	

BACK #5

(by itself)

Chakra

Back of sexual chakra—spleen chakra (see Front #4 & #5).

BACK #6

(by itself)

Physical

Male and female reproductive systems;
Hemorrhoids.

Chakra

Back of root chakra (see Front #4 & #5).

Oriental Medicine

At the base of the spine is the sacral bone. The name comes from the root word sacred. The medicine from India (Ayurveda, or the science of life) considers this to be the source of all the energetic conduits coursing through the body. This triangular shaped bone is the foundation of the spine; it should be treated for any problems involving the back from head to toe.

Notes

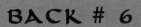

BACK # 6

CHAIR TREATMENT
- OTHER ➤

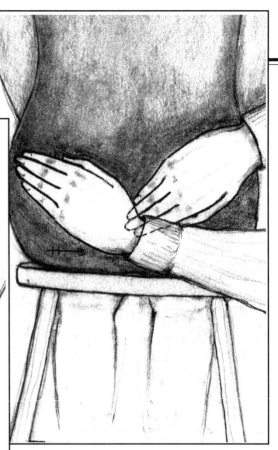

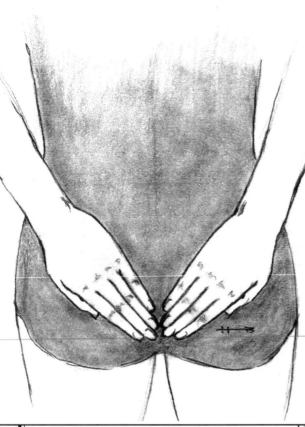

SELF TREATMENT ▲

TABLE TREATMENT
- OTHER ➤

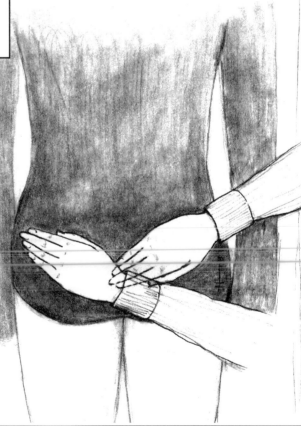

ALTERNATES

SELF TREATMENT
 - EAR ➤

SELF TREATMENT
 - TMJ ▲

SELF TREATMENT
 - SINUS ➤

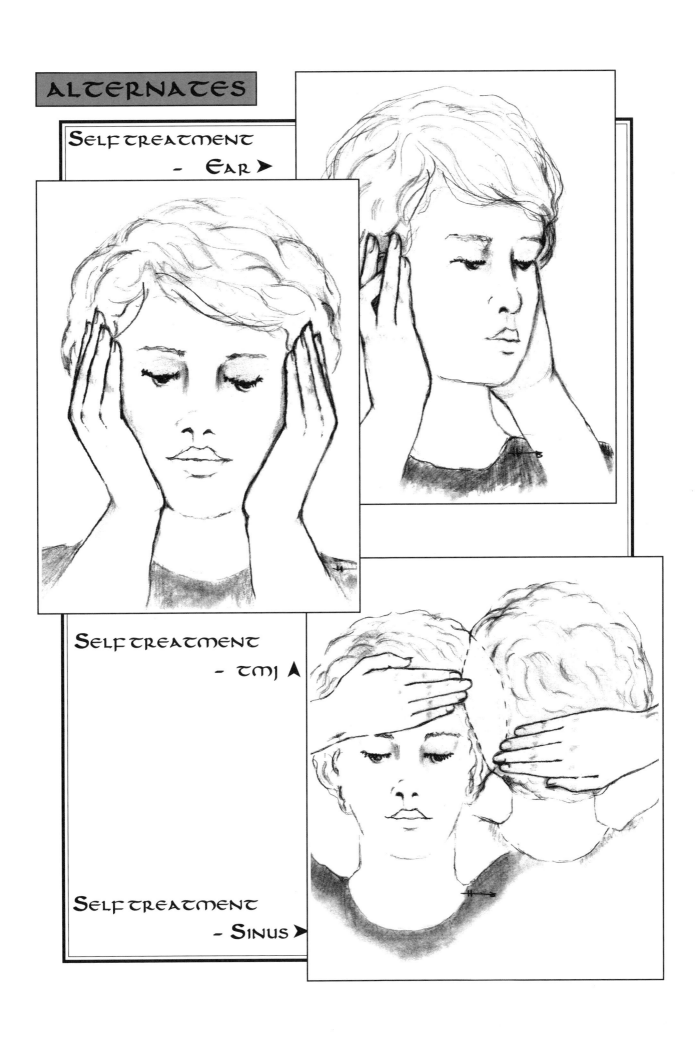

ALTERNATES

Table treatment
Other - Sinus ➤

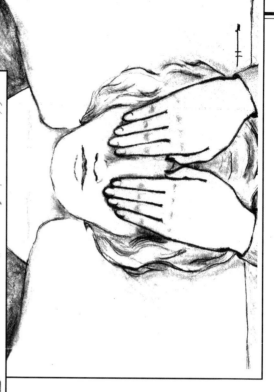

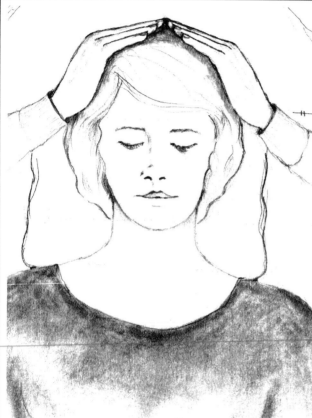

Chair treatment
Other - Head # 2 ▲

Table treatment
Other - Head # 2 ➤

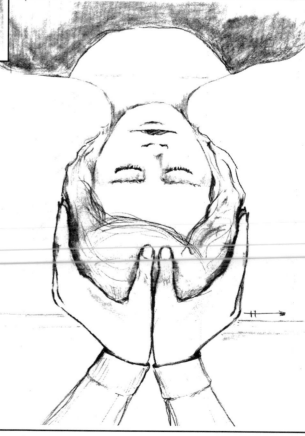

ALTERNATES

SELF TREATMENT - BREASTS ▶

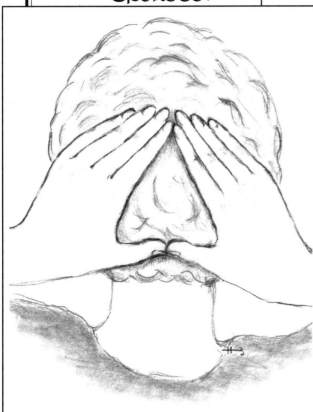

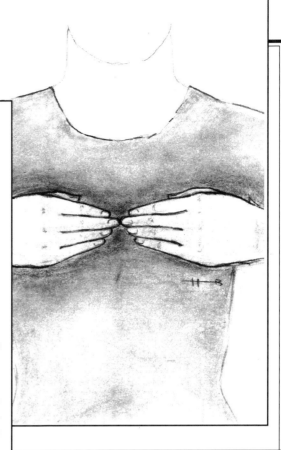

SELF TREATMENT - HEAD # 3 ▲

SELF TREATMENT - HEAD # 3 ▶

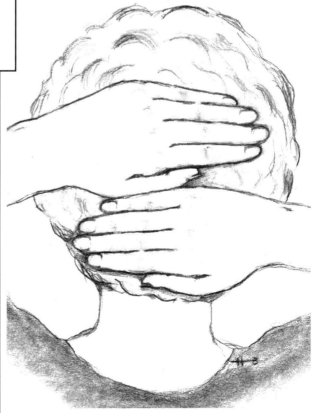

REIKI FINISH

CHAIR TREATMENT - OTHER ➤

SELF TREATMENT ▲

TABLE TREATMENT - OTHER ➤

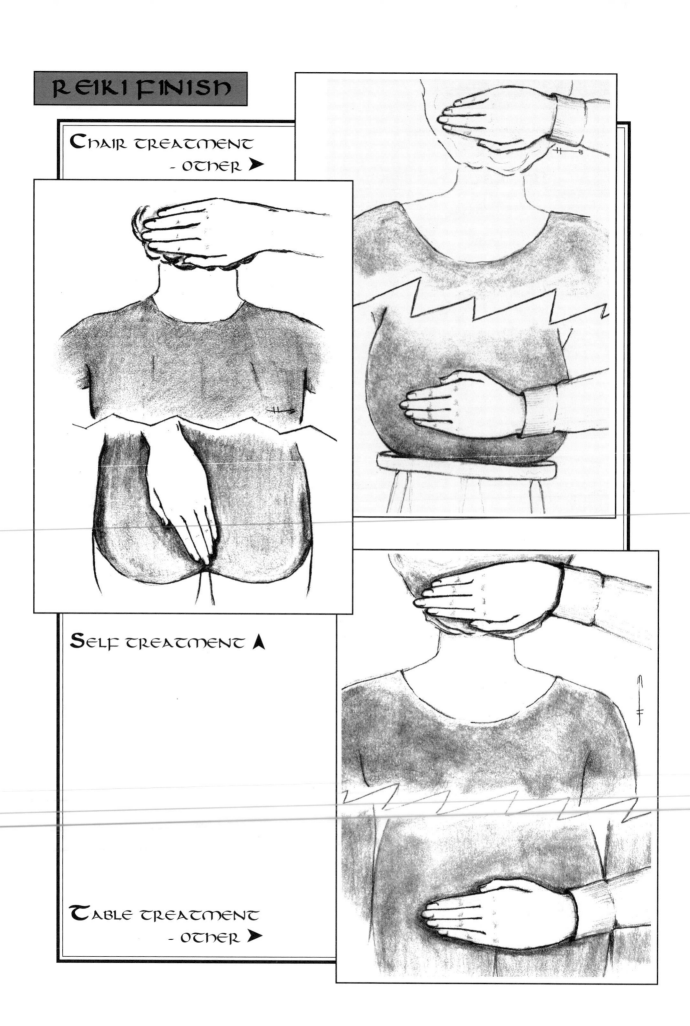

Placement of Hands

Place one hand on the base of the skull and one hand on the tailbone.

> This position runs energy up and down the spine, and gives a very effective and soothing finish to the Reiki treatment.
>
> At this point move away from your client very slowly because the auric field is greatly expanded at this time and too rapid a break with the energy would be startling (to yourself, also).

"If you have time for nothing else, do the Reiki finish! This is the most overall effective balancer I know of."
—Dr. George Avera, D.C.

Oriental Medicine

There is a parasympathetic nerve plexus at the tailbone. Treating this area with the base of the neck amplifies parasympathetic resonance within the system. This adds the vitalizing healing properties of Reiki to the biological connections of the nervous system, creating a deeply relaxed field of energy. This is a powerful combination and its healing power should not be underestimated.

Notes

NOTES

General Treatment Principles

BY WILLIAM MORRIS, O.M.D.

The **Law of Opposites** implies neurological polarization and crossover. It is commonly used in acupuncture. These principles may be used alone or combined with local treatment.

1. For that which is above, treat that which is below. For instance, treat the abdomen in cases of headaches;
2. Treat the opposite limb, leg to leg or arm to arm;
3. Treat the opposite limb contralaterally, left arm to right leg;
4. Treat same side arm and leg.

With right tennis elbow, also treat the following which correspond to the above principles (i.e., the right knee is treated for right elbow problems).

#1 treat lower extremities;
#2 add the left elbow;
#3 above, treat the left knee;
#4 above, the right knee.

The law of opposites also applies to the front and back of the torso. Better results will be achieved, for instance in a backache, by also treating the corresponding area on the front.

The Organ Clock is an ancient biorhythm system that has borne out through empirical observation and study. It may be useful in your treatments.

The organ clock of the Chinese can provide ideas as to where to focus treatment, based on the time of day the symptoms are aggravated. This can also be used to time treatments.

11 AM to 1 PM is Heart	11 PM to 1 AM is Gallbladder
1 PM to 3 PM is Small Intestine	1 AM to 3 AM is Liver
3 PM to 5 PM is Urinary Bladder	3 AM to 5 AM is Lung
5 PM to 7 PM is Kidney	5 AM to 7 AM is Large Intestine
7 PM to 9 PM is Pericardium	7 AM to 9 AM is Stomach
9 PM to 11 PM is Triple Warmer	9 AM to 11 AM is Spleen/Pancreas

The Triple Warmer is sometimes thought of as the connective tissue surrounding the abdominal cavity.

Obviously some of these times are not convenient. Through the law of opposites, we treat an organ energy that is active from 3 AM to 5 AM during the afternoon between 3 PM and 5 PM. In other words, we treat for the lung during the bladder time.

The body
the form
will be shaped
by the thought that
underlies it.

Vivekananda

Specific Treatments

For all of the treatments in this section, first give a full treatment (all 15 hand positions), then spend additional time on the positions listed here. Repeat this pattern daily for three days to start the healing process, and then as needed. This is the ideal way to give a treatment. I realize that many times you will not have the time to do a full treatment; do whatever you can.

While five minutes per position is appropriate to help someone in good health advance to optimal health, you cannot do too much or too little Reiki, and many, many hours of Reiki may be needed to facilitate a balance of the energy in a problem area. The three students I know whose broken arms were healed in less than ten days did not achieve this result with five-minute treatments. The people involved spent many hours holding their broken arm every day, they had family that gave them both "in person" and "absentee" treatments, and they were placed in our healing basket at the Center.

Reiki can be used for both "self treatment" and for the treatment of others. Some situations are best treated as "self treatments" because of the many hours of treatment needed. Other treatments are best done by another person because of the difficulty in reaching certain areas or because of the weakened state of the client. It is **always** recommended that people have Reiki to treat themselves between their sessions with a practitioner.

Our most amazing miracles usually occur with infants, accidents, and animals: infants because they are growing at such a rapid rate, accidents because the injury has not had a chance to get into cellular memory, and animals because they are so open to the energy.

It is helpful to look for the metaphysical causes for the dis-ease. I believe that most illnesses have metaphysical causes, and that only when we start working to heal the metaphysical causes will we facilitate a total healing on all levels.

For people with chronic problems it is **strongly** recommended that they, and all their close family members, have both First and Second Degree Reiki. It was not unusual for Madam Takata to actually move in with an ill person so she could treat extensively, and also so that the whole family could be given Reiki initiations and be able to treat the client.

Reiki is not meant to take the place of appropriate medical care. Please use common sense and seek whatever professional help may be needed, both with accidents and with chronic problems.

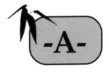

ABSCESS - Cover the abscess with a tissue and treat for 30 minutes (preferably twice daily), then treat the spleen to help cleanse and purify the blood. Treat until the abscess either breaks or is reabsorbed by the body.

ACCIDENTS - Treat directly on the injured area (especially if there is profuse bleeding) and on the adrenals, BACK 4, and over the solar plexus, FRONT 2 and 3. Get appropriate medical help immediately if it is needed.

ACNE - Treat directly on the area affected and also on HEAD 3, the spleen for blood purification, FRONT 4 and 5, and BACK 5 and 6 to help release toxins from the body faster. Frequently a colon cleanse program, when used in addition to Reiki treatments, will help to speed the healing process. Also consider treating for allergies.

ACUPRESSURE - See **ACUPUNCTURE**.

ACUPUNCTURE - When an acupuncturist has Reiki, the Reiki energy flows through the acupuncturist's hands, directly into, and through, the needles into the acupuncture point. Releases tend to be quicker and longer lasting than those from treatments without Reiki.

ADDICTIONS - I believe in an eclectic approach to any addiction, and Reiki should be an integral part of a program that includes abstinence, a Twelve Step Program (AA, OA, NA, etc.), counseling, vitamin and mineral therapy, and detoxing. Treat HEAD 3 for the old brain, FRONT 2 and 3 for the liver, FRONT 4 and 5, and BACK 5 and 6 for the release of toxins, and BACK 4 for the adrenals.

ADRENALS - Adrenalin overload as well as adrenal depletion or failure are all becoming common in our society today. Frequently, changes in lifestyle are required to overcome the problem. Treat on the adrenals, BACK 4, for as long and as often as possible, but a minimum of 30 minutes a day.

AGING - Reiki appears to slow down the aging process when used in conjunction with a healthy life style (diet, vitamin and mineral supplements, exercise, mental attitude, etc.). We frequently see people "young up" even during the class.

In addition to a daily full body treatment, treat HEAD 1, 2, 3, and FRONT 1. In addition, treat any areas that are causing current problems or discomfort.

AIDS - See **IMMUNE SYSTEM DISORDERS**.

ALLERGIES - Start by removing the cause of the allergy from the diet, or from the environment. Many people have unrecognized allergies to dairy products, wheat products, food additives, white sugar, and red meat. In the environment, some major troublemakers are dust, dog and cat dander, mattress mites, and "outgassing" from carpet, fabric, paints, etc. Treat HEAD 1 and 3 to clear the sinuses and to treat the old brain, FRONT 1 for the lungs, 2, and 3 for the digestion, 4, and 5 for detoxing, and at least 30 minutes daily on BACK 4 for the adrenals.

A.L.S. (AMYOTROPHIC LATERAL SCLEROSIS or "Lou Gehrig's Disease") - Full hands-on treatment, with Second Degree, AT LEAST twice daily with additional time on HEAD 1, 2 and 3, FRONT 1, and from top to bottom of the spine.

ALZHEIMER'S - Full hands-on treatment, with Second Degree, twice daily with extra time on HEAD 1, 2 and 3. Absentee treatments by family and friends can also help balance and reduce stress.

ANEMIA - Treat the spleen (left side above the waist), and the adrenals, BACK 4. Historically, a week's diet of the Reiki Slaw and Blood Replenisher has been suggested.

ANOREXIA NERVOSA - See **ADDICTIONS**.

ANXIETY - Treat HEAD 1, 2, and 3 to bring emotional balance, FRONT 2 and 3 for centering and BACK 4 for the adrenals.

ARC - See **IMMUNE SYSTEM DISORDER**. The designation of AIDS-Related Complex is rarely used now that the definition of AIDS has been broadened.

ARMS, LEGS, HANDS, AND FEET - Treat any muscle or joint problem directly on the area of need, sandwiching it between your hands either top to bottom or side to side.

ARTHRITIS - See **AUTO-IMMUNE SYSTEM DISORDERS**.

ASTHMA - see **ALLERGIES**. Second Degree hands-on treatments are necessary. After the full body treatment, you must also add 30 minutes of treatments on each side of the pleura, the side of the lungs, by placing both of your hands on the side of the torso above the waist while the person is lying on his or her opposite side. Treat for 21 consecutive days; if there is a break in the number of days, it is necessary to start back at Day 1, and do the FULL 21 days.

AUTO-IMMUNE SYSTEM DISORDERS (Arthritis, Graves Disease, Pernicious Anemia, Lupus, etc.) - Frequently it is necessary to take a close look at one's diet. Many arthritic type problems are helped by eliminating certain foods that are toxic to the person in discomfort. Many people also get relief from treatments and herbal supplements given by an Oriental Medical Doctor/Licensed Acupuncturist. Treat HEAD 3 for the old brain, FRONT 5 for the bladder, BACK 3 for the kidneys, and BACK 4 for the adrenals. Spend extra time on any painful or swollen areas to break up the calcium deposits. Drink ample liquids to flush toxins from the system.

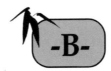

BACKACHES - For acute pain, treat directly on the problem area. For chronic pain, start at the base of the skull and treat all of the way down the spine to the tailbone (be sure to not miss any of the spine). Also give extra time to FRONT 5 and 6. Attempt to determine the metaphysical cause of the condition and treat accordingly.

BALDNESS - Treat directly over the bald spots for as long as possible each day. This is best done by another person since many hours of treatment are required. However, Reiki treatment HAS been known to regenerate hair growth for many people. Massage vitamin E oil into the scalp each evening, and shampoo the head each morning with a gentle shampoo.

BED WETTING - Strengthen the bladder by treating FRONT 5 and BACK 6.

BEE STINGS - Start by removing the stinger if possible. Gently suck on the wound for about a minute, spitting out the venom frequently (do NOT do this if you have any type of sore in your mouth or on your lips). Place one hand on the wound and the other either above the wound (toward the heart), or on the opposite side if the wound is on an arm or leg. Treat for at least 20 to 30 minutes. If the person's reaction is extreme, also treat the lymphatic system—both sides of the neck, under the arms, thymus area, and groin.

BELL'S PALSY - Treat HEAD positions 1, 2, 3, 4, then also treat the jaws, cheeks, mouth, and behind the ears.

BLEEDING - Cover the wound with a clean cloth and treat directly on the wound if possible. If you are concerned about exposure to the blood then cover the cloth with a plastic covering.

BLISTERS - see **BURNS**.

BLOOD PRESSURE - Balance both high and low blood pressure by treating HEAD 3 and 4, and FRONT 1. Yogic breathing, guided visualizations, and biofeedback are also extremely helpful.

BOILS - See **ABSCESS**.

BRAIN INJURY or TUMORS - Spend as much time as possible on all four head positions, and add hand positions on each side of the head, if called for. Remember that with head injuries there is often damage on the side of the head OPPOSITE the injury.

BREASTS - For any breast problem (male or female), lumps, abscesses, cancer, etc., treatment should be directly on the breast area. Unless the person is your partner, it is illegal to give such a treatment; it is therefore recommended that the person get Reiki for themselves. The treatment consists of as much time as possible directly on the breasts, and at least 20 minutes on FRONT 5.

BROKEN BONES - Do not treat directly on the break until AFTER it has been set. Instead treat above and below the break. As soon as the break has been set, treat through the cast for as many hours as possible with Second Degree.

BRONCHITIS - Same as treatment for **ALLERGIES**.

BULIMIA - See **ADDICTIONS**.

BURNS - Place hands directly over, NOT ON, the burned area. Treat for 15 minutes or until after the pain goes away, then treat BACK 4 for the adrenals.

BURSITIS - See **ARTHRITIS**.

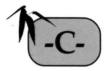

CALLUSES and CORNS - Sometimes the cause is a misalignment. Suggest a chiropractic checkup of the spine, legs and feet. Treat the spine, hips, and the area of the foot that is involved.

CANCER - see **IMMUNE SYSTEM DISORDERS**.

CANDIDA ALBICANS - Daily treatments with extra time on HEAD 3, BACK 4, and spleen.

CARBUNCLE - See **ABSCESS**.

CARPAL TUNNEL - See **TENDONITIS**.

CATARACT - See **EYES**.

CEREBRAL PALSY - Daily treatments are necessary with extra time spent on treating HEAD 2 and 3, FRONT 1, 2 and 3, and BACK 3.

CHEMOTHERAPY - Full daily Second Degree treatments with extra time on spleen, liver, and adrenals.

CHILDBIRTH - Treat as much as possible during the pregnancy, giving the mother full treatments and covering the entire abdominal area. During labor, have as many people as possible doing absentee treatments on both mother and child. Treat the mother hands-on during the labor process on BACK 5 and 6, the lower back, and the total abdominal area, FRONT 3 down through 5, with as many added hand positions as needed.

CHIROPRACTIC - When Reiki is used in conjunction with spinal or other adjustments, the adjustments are faster and tend to hold longer.

CHRONIC FATIGUE SYNDROME (CFS) - See **IMMUNE SYSTEM DISORDER.**

CIRRHOSIS OF THE LIVER - See **LIVER.**

CIRCULATION - Begin with HEAD 3 and 4, then FRONT 1 and 5. If you are treating yourself or your partner, you may also treat the groin area by placing the middle finger of one hand on the large artery going to the leg (the soft spot just behind the tendon that goes from the torso down into the leg), and the other hand on FRONT 4. Circulation in the hands is improved by having Reiki for yourself and running the energy through them by giving lots of treatments.

COLDS - Treat twice daily for three consecutive days giving a full treatment each time, then extra time on FRONT 1 and 5. In addition, for head colds spend extra time on HEAD 1, 2 and 3, and for chest colds spend extra time on HEAD 4, FRONT 2, BACK 1 and 2 and on both sides of the rib cage (the pleura).

COLIC - Hold the baby so one hand treats the stomach area and the other hand treats the back. Treat until gas is released and the baby is able to go to sleep. Often one very extended treatment has been known to clear up the problem.

COMA - Spend extra time on HEAD 1, 2 and 3, on FRONT 1, 2 and 3, and on BACK 4. Team treatments are especially helpful, and absentee treatments are also effective.

COMPULSIVE OVEREATING - See **OBESITY** and **ADDICTIONS.**

CONGENITAL DEFECTS - Birth defects should be treated intrauterine if possible and require full body treatments as quickly after birth as possible. The problem is seldom cured, but improvements have occurred when treatment was begun early in the pregnancy. It is also helpful for the child to have First Degree so that whenever they touch themselves they are running the energy.

CONSTIPATION - Treat HEAD 3, FRONT 4 and 5, and BACK 5 and 6.

COUGHS - See **COLDS.** Spend extra time on the diaphragm, FRONT 2.

CRAMPS - See **MENSTRUAL PROBLEMS.**

CUTS - Treat immediately to stop the bleeding and to seal the cut. Clean, bandage and continue to treat. Get medical care if stitches are necessary and continue treating as much as possible to speed up the healing of the wound.

CYSTIC FIBROSIS - Daily full treatments with extra time on HEAD 3, FRONT 1 and 2, BACK 1 and 2 and both pleuras.

CYSTITIS - Treat FRONT 5, BACK 6 and spleen.

CYSTS - See **ABSCESS**.

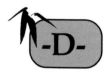

DEAFNESS - See **EARS**.

DEATH AND DYING - See **TRANSITION PROCESS**.

DENTAL AND GUM PROBLEMS - Treat directly over the problem area (directly in the mouth if self treatment). Homeopathic remedies are very helpful in the healing process of dental and gum problems.

DEPRESSION - See **EMOTIONAL DISORDERS**.

DETACHED RETINA - Spend as much time as possible on HEAD 1. Also treat HEAD 2 and 3.

DIABETES - If the client is on insulin be sure they keep very close watch on insulin needs since there will usually be a dramatic drop in insulin requirements. Treat HEAD 3, FRONT 2 (minimum of 30 minutes) and 3, and BACK 4. If there is a problem, or a potential problem, with diabetic blindness treat HEAD 1, 2, 3, and FRONT 5 for women (ovaries), or BACK 6 for men (prostate).

DIALYSIS - Reiki can be used to lessen the cramping while on a dialysis machine by treating directly on the muscles involved. Daily Second Degree treatments are needed with extra time spent on the liver, spleen, FRONT 4 and 5, and BACK 3, 5 and 6.

DIARRHEA - Spend time on FRONT 4 and 5, and BACK 5 and 6.

DIGESTIVE DISORDERS - Start with HEAD 3 then proceed to FRONT 2 and 3, FRONT 4 and 5, and BACK 5 and 6. Papaya enzymes or hydrochloric acid supplements are very helpful for many people.

DIVERTICULOSIS - See **DIARRHEA**.

DIZZINESS - See **EQUILIBRIUM PROBLEMS**.

DREAM RECALL - HEAD 3 is the position to treat as you are falling asleep at night. Keep a dream journal beside your bed and write in it immediately upon waking up.

DROPPED FOOT - This special hand position can be used only on your partner for legal reasons. Have your partner lie on his or her back with legs spread apart, knees bent slightly. Then place your middle finger on the groin area where the leg joins the body, and the other hand on FRONT 5 on the same side of the body. Proceed on to treating the calf, the ankle and the foot by sandwiching each area between your hands.

DRUG ADDICTION - See **ADDICTIONS**.

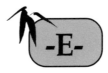

EARS - Gently place the middle fingers directly into the ear and the other fingers close in, both in front of the ears and behind them. If the ear is too tender for the fingers to be placed in the ear, then "cup" the hands over the ears. Cupping is less direct and will take longer.

EDEMA - Fluid retention can be relieved by treating HEAD 3, FRONT 4 and 5, and BACK 3 and 4. Check with your health food store or holistic pharmacy for natural diuretics.

EMOTIONAL DISORDERS - HEAD 2 is the primary treatment position. It is beneficial to also give extra time to HEAD 1 and 3, FRONT 2 and 3, and BACK 4. Use of the Second Degree mental, emotional, and addictive treatment is strongly recommended.

EMPHYSEMA - see **ALLERGIES**. Treatment is necessary for 30 consecutive days. If anything interferes with the total 30-day treatment you must start back at Day number 1 of the treatment series.

ENERGIZING / QUICK PICKER-UPPER - Place one hand on the Solar Plexus and the other on the navel.

EPILEPSY - Treat HEAD 2. Begin the treatment at the onset of the seizure, if at all possible, and continue for as long as possible.

EPSTEIN-BARR VIRUS - See **IMMUNE SYSTEM DISORDERS**.

EQUILIBRIUM PROBLEMS - HEAD 2 is the primary position, however, also treat HEAD 1 and 3, and both ears.

EYES - Treat HEAD 1, 2 and 3 so that both eyes and both eye-stems are completely treated. Frequently there are also related glandular problems in need of treatment. This is the treatment for cataracts, glaucoma, near-sightedness or far-sightedness, and infections.

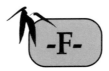

FASTING - Twice daily treatments will help replenish your vital life force energy and speed up the cleansing process. Spend extra time on HEAD 3, FRONT 4 and 5, and BACK 3, 5 and 6.

FATIGUE - Treat HEAD 1 and 3, FRONT 3, and BACK 4. Falling asleep with one or both hands on HEAD 3 will speed up the balancing process.

FEET - See **ARMS**.

FEVER - Fevers can usually be broken with a full treatment and extra treatment time on HEAD 3 and 4, and on BACK 4.

FIBROMYALGIA SYNDROME - Daily full treatments, plus a hand on HEAD 3 before going to sleep. Spend extra time on knees, elbows, upper thigh on the back of the leg, and on the spleen.

FLU - See **COLDS**.

FOOD - By holding your hands slightly above your food before you start to eat you will make it more harmonious with your body.

FOOD POISONING - Spend extra time on FRONT 2, 3, 4 and 5, and on BACK 3, 5 and 6.

FRACTURES - See **BROKEN BONES**.

FROSTBITE - Treat immediately on the affected areas and on BACK 4 for the adrenals. Afterward give a full body treatment as soon as possible.

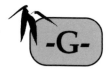

GALL BLADDER - Treat the right side of both FRONT 2 and 3, and the right side of BACK 4. Frequently a "glug-glug" sound will be both heard and felt when treating directly over the gall bladder as it releases.

GALLSTONES - See **GALL BLADDER**. A very lengthy treatment or several shorter treatments will frequently pulverize the stones so they may be passed.

GAS - See **DIARRHEA**.

GLAUCOMA - See **EYES**.

GOUT - see **ARTHRITIS**. Also consider eating cherries or drinking cherry juice.

GROUNDING - Hold soles of the feet, then place one hand on the Solar Plexus and one on the navel, or place one hand on the top of the head and the other on the Solar Plexus.

GUMS - See **DENTAL AND GUM PROBLEMS**.

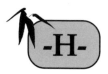

HAIR - See **BALDNESS**.

HANDS - See **ARMS**.

HANGOVER - Head 1, 2 and 3, FRONT 2 and 3, and BACK 4.

HEAD INJURIES - See **BRAIN INJURY**.

HEADACHE - MIGRAINE - Treat FRONT 1, 2, 3 and 4, then 30 minutes on FRONT 5 for women, or BACK 6 for men, since there appears to be a link between migraines, and ovaries or prostate. Next treat HEAD 1, 2 and 3. A minimum of three consecutive days of treatment is recommended.

HEADACHE - TENSION - Treat HEAD 1, 2, 3 and 4, FRONT 2 and 3 to detox the liver, Front 5 and 6 to speed up the release of toxins, and BACK 1 for shoulder tension. Try to remove the cause of the tension and do a neck and shoulder Release. Chiropractic adjustments are frequently called for and regular massages can help to keep the body's tension level down. Vitamin B Complex is noted for stress reduction and for replacing the vitamins depleted by stress.

HEADACHE - TOXINS - See **HEADACHE - TENSION**.

HEART ATTACK - Get professional help immediately, then place both hands over the heart/diaphragm area (at center on left side of the body). There will often be a release of gas, sounding and feeling like "glug," after which you can progress to FRONT 1, 2 and BACK 4 for the adrenals.

HEARTBURN - Treat HEAD 3, FRONT 2 and 3.

HEMATOMA - Be sure to first do a full body treatment, then place hands directly over the swollen area. Blood is re-absorbed by the body.

HEMOPHILIA - Treat HEAD 3 for the old brain, and FRONT 2 and 3 for the pancreas.

HEMORRHAGE - Get professional help immediately. Place one hand over the problem area and the other over the heart. It is always best to protect yourself with latex so you are not directly exposed to someone else's blood.

HEMORRHOIDS - Treat with a variation of BACK 6: put the middle finger directly over the anal opening, and the other hand across the base of the spine. Treat for 30 minutes. For legal reasons this treatment must ONLY be done on yourself or your partner. There is a Homeopathic Remedy for piles that, when used in conjunction with Reiki treatments, is extremely effective.

HEPATITIS - See **LIVER**.

HERNIA - Treat directly on the hernia after the projection has been placed back into the opening.

HERPES - Treat to reduce stress and treat directly on the affected area for as long as possible.

HIATAL HERNIA - Treat directly over the diaphragm, FRONT 2. An old treatment that is very effective used with your Reiki is to drink a glass of water, hold your hands above your head, and jump up and down several times.

HICCUPS - Have the client lie down with arms stretched over his or her head. Place one hand on the base of the sternum (breast bone), and the other directly below it. To treat yourself, place both hands in this same position, one hand above the other on the sternum. Treat until the hiccups are gone.

HIGH BLOOD PRESSURE - Primary treatment is HEAD 4 to treat the carotid arteries, but you should also treat the old brain, HEAD 3. Guided visualization and biofeedback are excellent modalities for lowering blood pressure. Also carefully check the diet.

HIV POSITIVE - See **IMMUNE SYSTEM DISORDERS**.

HOMEOPATHY - Reiki is one of the few energy systems that can be used safely with Homeopathy without neutralizing the remedies.

HYPERTENSION - See **HIGH BLOOD PRESSURE**.

HYPNOSIS - Many hypnotherapists incorporate the balancing power of Reiki as part of the process used to take a client "to level." Simply keeping a hand on the client's arm during the process is usually adequate. The feedback I get is that the clients go deeper, faster when Reiki is used.

HYPOGLYCEMIA - Daily full treatments with extra time on HEAD 3, FRONT 2 (minimum of 30 minutes), and 3, and BACK 4.

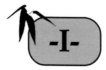

IMMUNE SYSTEM DISORDERS - This covers any breakdown of the immune system such as Lupus, Chronic Fatigue Syndrome (CFS), Epstein-Barr Virus (EBV), HIV+, AIDS, Cancer, Crohn's Disease, etc. Treat HEAD POSITIONS 2, 3 and 4, FRONT 1 and 5, BACK 4, spleen, and any specific area involved.

IMPOTENCE - Treat HEAD 3, FRONT 5, BACK 4 and 6 for the adrenals. If you are treating yourself or your partner then treat directly over the prostate.

INDIGESTION - See **DIGESTIVE DISORDERS**.

INFECTIONS - Treat HEAD 3, BACK 4, on the left side for the spleen, and directly on the infection.

INFLUENZA - See **COLDS**.

INSECT BITES - See **BEE STINGS**.

INSOMNIA - See **SLEEP DISORDERS**.

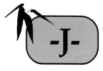

JAUNDICE - See **LIVER**.

JOINTS - See **ARTHRITIS**.

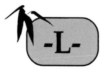

LARYNGITIS - Treat directly on the throat. Look for what the metaphysical cause might be—for example, fear of saying something, inability to speak up for oneself, holding back on expressing oneself, etc.

LEARNING AND MEMORY - The primary position is HEAD 2; however, time should also be spent on HEAD 3 and 4 and FRONT 3. Research has shown that quiet peaceful music can help retention.

LEGS - See **ARMS**.

LIVER - To completely cover the liver, which is on the right side of the body, you will start with both hands, one above the other, to the right of the front center line of the body. Continue working your way around the body until you reach the center of the back. This is a very lengthy treatment and is in addition to, not instead of, a full treatment.

LUPUS - See **IMMUNE SYSTEM DISORDERS**.

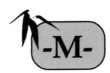

MALE MENOPAUSE / MID-LIFE CRISIS -See **MENOPAUSE**.
This is probably related to hormonal shifts in a man just as it is in a woman.

MANIC-DEPRESSIVE (BIPOLAR) ILLNESS - See **EMOTIONAL DISORDERS**.

MASSAGE - Start a massage by doing 5 minutes of Reiki in HEAD 1 or 2 to tap into the energy. Continue by doing your usual massage, then end the massage with 5 minutes on the soles of the feet. Reiki is NOT a massage, but as you can see, it can be used with and enhances any massage modality.

MEASLES - Do a full body treatment immediately for adults but wait 24 hours before treating children. Spend extra time on HEAD 1.

MEDITATION - Reiki is a wonderful adjunct to any form of meditation you might practice. Place your hands in an appropriate place, depending upon your type of meditation, such as over the heart, on the throat, over the eyes or in the ears—or simply turn your hands over so that your palms rest on your knees.

MEMORY - See **LEARNING and MEMORY**.

MENOPAUSE - Treat HEAD 3 for the old brain, FRONT 2 and 3 on the right side for the liver, FRONT 5 for the ovaries, BACK 4 for the adrenals, and BACK 6 for the back of the ovaries. Oriental Medicine has many wonderful herbs to help with menopause and acupuncture needles can release many blockages that cause problems. I personally recommend this natural approach.

MENSTRUAL PROBLEMS - Begin treatment 4 to 5 days before the onset of menses and continue throughout the period. Treat HEAD 3, FRONT 5, and BACK 6. Frequently, taking calcium-magnesium supplements and an herbal diuretic will assist in alleviating the pain.

MIGRAINE - See **HEADACHE**.

MOLES and WARTS - Treat by pinching gently between the fingers as often as possible and they will usually dry up and drop off.

MOTION SICKNESS - This is an inner ear problem, so the primary treatment areas are HEAD 2, 3 and 4, along with FRONT 2.

MOUTH SORES - See **DENTAL AND GUM PROBLEMS**.

MULTIPLE SCLEROSIS - Full Second Degree treatments twice daily are recommended, with extra time on HEAD 2 and 3, FRONT 2 and 3, and on the spine from top to bottom, and the Reiki Finish. Clients should have Reiki and be taught to keep their hands on themselves whenever possible.

MUMPS - Do a full body treatment immediately on adults, but wait 24 hours before treating a child. Extra time should be spent on the spleen and areas of concentration of lymph glands (throat, underarms, and groin), with 30 minutes spent treating the ovaries or testicles (only on yourself or your partner, of course, for legal reasons).

MUSCULAR DYSTROPHY - Full Second Degree treatments twice daily are recommended with extra time on HEAD 1, 2 and 3, FRONT 1, 2 and 3, and BACK 2 and 3. Clients should have Reiki and be taught to keep their hands on themselves whenever possible.

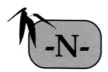

NASAL POLYPS - Place hand gently around the nose (no pressure needed) as long as possible for several treatments. There is a Homeopathic Remedy that is great when used with your Reiki.

NAUSEA - Treat HEAD 3, FRONT 2 and 3. Be prepared for possible vomiting since the body sometimes detoxes rapidly with Reiki.

NERVOUSNESS - See **EMOTIONAL DISORDERS**.

NOSEBLEED - Client should be placed at a 45 degree angle with an ice bag on the back of the neck. Cup your hand around the nose with your thumb on one side and fingers balled up on the other to close off the nasal opening. Place your other hand on the base of the skull.

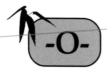

OBESITY (OVEREATING, OVERWEIGHT) - See **ADDICTIONS**. In addition, treat HEAD 3 for old brain and 4 for thyroid, FRONT 2, 3 for liver and digestion, and FRONT 4 and 5 for detoxing. Frequently a colon cleanse is helpful, and self-esteem issues probably need to be worked on and healed.

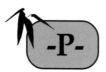

PAIN - There is a soft spot on the top of the shoulders next to the bone (the bra strap spot), that is a major endorphin-releasing spot for the body. Treat this spot for pain anywhere in the body because endorphins are a natural morphine the body produces (morphine is a pain-killer).

PARALYSIS - Full body treatments twice daily, extra time on HEAD 3, BACK 4, and on the affected areas. Clients should have Reiki and be taught to keep their hands on themselves whenever possible, and to do full body treatments with the Second Degree Absentee technique several times daily.

PARKINSON'S DISEASE - Full treatments twice daily are necessary with extra time spent on HEAD 1, 2, 3, and 4, FRONT 2, BACK 4, and both hands.

PAST LIFE RECALL - See **HYPNOSIS**.

PHOBIAS - See **EMOTIONAL DISORDERS**.

PLEURISY - See **COLDS**.

PNEUMONIA - Do the total treatment with client lying on his or her back with the head and upper torso slightly elevated. Spend extra time on HEAD 1, 2, 3 and 4, FRONT 1, 2 and 3, top of the shoulders (the gateway to the lungs), and by slipping the hands under the body treat BACK 2 and 4. In non-crisis situations, treat daily until the fever breaks (usually 4 or 5 days). In crisis situations treat continuously if possible until the fever breaks (could take 4 to 5 hours). Team and absentee treatments are strongly recommended wherever possible.

PREGNANCY - See **CHILDBIRTH**.

PREMENSTRUAL SYNDROM (PMS) - See **MENSTRUAL PROBLEMS**.

PREVENTIVE HEALTH CARE - When full-body treatments are used on a daily basis, Reiki helps to create a level of optimal health that serves to ward off potential physical and emotional problems.

PROSTATE - Primary treatment position is directly on the prostate gland. This can only be done on yourself or your partner for legal reasons. Also treat HEAD 4 for the thyroid gland.

PSORIASIS - Daily full treatments with extra time on HEAD 3 and directly on the scaley areas.

PSYCHOSOMATIC ILLNESSES - Daily full body treatments with extra time on HEAD 3.

PYORRHEA - See **DENTAL and GUM PROBLEMS**. On ten consecutive days treat for 30 minutes on the mouth and 10 minutes on the spleen in addition to full body treatment.

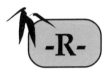

RADIATION - Twice daily do full treatments with extra time on the spleen and on the area exposed to the radiation. Epsom salts baths help to draw out the toxins.

RASH - Treat directly on the problem area. Check for allergies or other possible causes. A change of diet may be called for.

REFLEXOLOGY - Reiki goes directly into the reflex points and facilitates quick releases that last longer than they do without Reiki.

RELAXATION - See **STRESS REDUCTION**.

RHEUMATISM - see **ARTHRITIS**.

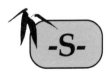

SCARS - Treat directly over the scar tissue as often and as long as possible. Very little can be expected if the scar is over two years old. Fasting is considered by some to help dissolve scars.

SCHIZOPHRENIA - See **EMOTIONAL DISORDERS**.

SCIATIC NERVE PROBLEMS - Start with the fingers of both hands touching the spine, with the upper hand touching, but below, the waist. Be sure that as you work your way down the hip and leg that you overlap hand positions and do not miss even a fraction of an inch of space. As you get to the lower part of the hip, start angling out so that you will be treating the upper-outer quadrant of the leg. Work your way down the entire leg and end the treatment in the arch of the foot. Draw the energy out and away from the body when you are finished. This treatment will take from 1 to 2 hours to complete, is extremely difficult to do on yourself, but is very effective.

SCLERODERMA - Daily full body treatments with extra time over the hardening areas.

SENILITY - Extra time spent on HEAD 1, 2 and 3, FRONT 1 for the heart, and BACK 4 for the adrenals.

SEXUAL PROBLEMS - Spend extra time on HEAD 3, FRONT 5 and BACK 6. Treat directly on the vaginal area or the prostate if giving self treatment or working on your partner (with their permission, of course). If emotions are involved, treat FRONT 1 for the heart.

SEXUALLY TRANSMITTED DISEASES - In addition to full body treatments, extra time should be spent on the spleen, the lymph glands (throat, underarms, and groin) and BACK 4 for adrenals, and if you are working on yourself or your partner, you can treat directly on the sexual organs.

SHINGLES - After completing a full treatment, place one hand below the sternum (breastbone) and the other on the left shoulder blade and treat for 10 to 15 minutes, then treat all affected areas. Because of extreme sensitivity, it may be necessary to treat above the affected areas, instead of touching them.

SHOCK - Get professional help immediately. Omit a full treatment. Go directly to HEAD 2 and 3, FRONT 3 for the solar plexus, and then BACK 4 for the adrenals.

SICKLE-CELL ANEMIA - Daily full treatments with extra time on spleen, liver, heart, lungs, joints and the full length of the arms and legs. Clients will need Reiki for themselves because of the extensive treatments needed.

SINUS PROBLEMS - Treat HEAD 1, 2 and 3 to get all sinus cavities, then FRONT 1, BACK 1 and 2. Check for allergies.

SLEEP APNEA - Spend extended time on HEAD 3.

SLEEP DISORDERS - Give a short treatment to HEAD 2, then place one hand on HEAD 3 and the other on the solar plexus. Support your arms with pillows and try to fall asleep with your hands in this position. A mental, emotional and addictive treatment with Second Degree is highly recommended. Celestial Seasoning's "Sleepytime Tea," or chamomile tea, is very good for relaxation, and I've had very positive feedback regarding use of my tape, "Color Breathing and Affirmations."

SMOKING - See **ADDICTIONS**.

SNAKE BITE - Use appropriate first aid by placing a tight wrap between the wound and the heart. Place one hand on the wound and the other over blood vessels between the wound and the heart. If other Reiki Therapists are available, have them treat the entire lymphatic system, neck, underarms, and groin (if legal), and BACK 4 for the adrenals.

SPRAIN - Treat directly on the sprain as quickly as possible after the injury and for as long as possible.

STRESS REDUCTION - Reiki is one of the best tools for stress reduction on the planet today. By giving oneself daily treatments, it is easier to handle situations as they come up without becoming stressed out over them.

STROKE - Get professional help immediately. Full treatments twice daily are recommended for a minimum of 4 days, with extra time spent on HEAD 2, 3 and 4 (at least 1 hour), FRONT 1, 2 and 3, and BACK 4. Treat arms and/or legs if they are affected.

STUTTERING - See **EMOTIONAL DISORDERS**.

SUNBURN - See **BURNS**.

SURGERY - Treat for as many days as possible before the surgery. Treat the person, the doctors, and the nurses involved during the surgery with Second Degree Absentee Treatments, and treat extensively after the surgery, both in person and using absentee treatment.

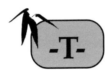

TACHYCARDIA - Treat directly over the heart.

TENDONITIS - Treat directly on the area for at least 30 minutes daily. Check to see what repetitive motion is being made with the arm or leg, and work to change to a different movement.

TENNIS ELBOW - See **TENDONITIS**.

THYROID PROBLEMS - The thyroid is a Master Gland and as such must be functioning properly for the whole body to function properly. Because of the tie-in between the thyroid and the adrenal glands, it is necessary to treat both FRONT 4 and BACK 4.

TIC DOULOUREUX - Daily treatments on HEAD 1, 2 and 3, under the chin, over the cheek/jaw area and over the lips. For the first few days do not touch the face, as it is far too sensitive, but treat slightly above it.

TINNITUS (Ringing in the ears) - See **EARS**.

TMJ (Tempero-Mandibular Joint Dysfunction) - Treat on both sides of the head in front of the ears, and at the base of the skull. Many chiropractors and some dentists work effectively with TMJ.

TONSILLITIS - Treat HEAD 3 and 4, under the lower jaw, for 15 to 20 minutes, and on the spleen.

TRANSITION PROCESS - Reiki offers loved ones, and those who are working professionally with people in the death and dying process, to be able to be supportive during the process rather than having to sit by helplessly. Treat over FRONT 1 for the heart, and use the Second Degree Absentee Treatment for the person in transition, the caregivers, and those affected to ease the journey for all. Birthing is also a transition process. As one grows on the Spiritual Path it becomes easier to see the cycles we go through as we grow and change, and grow and change while reaching for enlightenment.

TUMORS - Treat directly on the tumor, for as much time as possible, in addition to daily full body treatments. Several people have taped their hands over the tumor while sleeping to get hours of treatment and have had profound results.

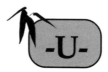

ULCERS - Use full Reiki treatments daily to lower the stress level, try to remove stressors from your life, and treat directly over the painful area as often as possible and for as long a time as possible.

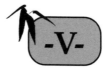

VAGINITIS - See **SEXUAL PROBLEMS**.

VARICOSE VEINS - See **CIRCULATION**. Additional time should be spent directly on the problem veins.

VENEREAL DISEASES - See **SEXUALLY TRANSMITTED DISEASES**.

VOMITING - See **NAUSEA**.

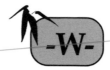

WHIPLASH - Treat HEAD 1, 2, 3 and 4. Treat also on the sides and back of the neck for 30 minutes or more.

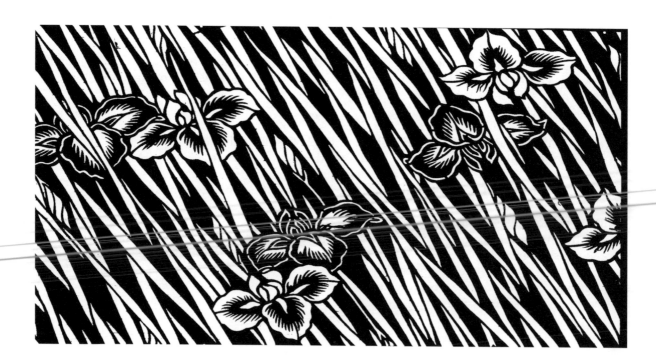

Appendix A

REIKI HEALING:
A PHYSIOLOGIC PERSPECTIVE AND IMPLICATIONS FOR NURSING

A Thesis by
Wendy S. Wetzel, RN, BSN

ABSTRACT

Purpose

Healing therapies which employ touch and are based on the premise of a human energy field are gaining in popularity and support throughout our culture. Reiki, an ancient healing art, is one such modality. But Reiki has not yet been submitted to close scientific scrutiny. The purpose of this study is to examine the effects of Reiki healing on human hemoglobin and hematocrit levels.

Procedures

Using Dr. Dolores Krieger's protocol for hemoglobin studies within the context of Therapeutic Touch, the hemoglobin and hematocrit levels of forty-eight adults participating in First Degree Reiki Training were measured. Demographics and motivation were also examined. An untreated control group was used to document the changes in hemoglobin and hematocrit under normal circumstances.

Findings

Findings were analyzed through the use of a t-test and revealed a statistically significant change between the pre- and post-training hemoglobin and hematocrit levels of the participants at the $p > 0.01$ level. The comparable control group, not experiencing the training, demonstrated no changes in hemoglobin or hematocrit levels. Further research is necessary to clarify the physiologic effects of touch healing.

Conclusions

This study documented one measurable physiologic effect of Reiki. The data lends support to the basic premise of energy transmission between individuals for the purposes of healing, balancing, and increasing wellness.

Chair: Leonide L. Martin, RN, Dr.P.H.
         M.S. Program: Nursing
         Sonoma State University

EXCERPTS FROM DEMOGRAPHICS

Sex, Race and Age

In the experimental group of 48, there were 14 males (29.2 percent) and 34 females (70.8 percent). Caucasians dominated the group (43 participants = 89.5 percent), with three Hispanics (6.3 percent), one Asian (2 percent), and one Filipino (2 percent). The mean age for the group was 40 years, 4 months, with a range of 24 to 69 years.

Education

This group is well educated. One-half (24) had obtained a bachelor's degree or more. The mean educational achievement was between an associate and bachelor's degrees, with slightly over three years of college. Thirteen participants (27 percent) have completed a post-graduate degree, nine (18.7 percent) have bachelor's degrees. No one area of study was predominant: education was listed by four subjects (one at the bachelor's level, and three at the master's level): nursing, business, psychology, theology, behavioral science, and medicine were noted by two respondents; other listed majors (architecture, occupational therapy, physical therapy, history, religion, and health sciences) were noted once each. Several respondents did not indicate a major area of study. Two subjects (4 percent) indicated they had some postgraduate work but did not indicate the area.

Of the remainder, five (10.4 percent) had high school diplomas, twelve (25 percent) had one or two years of college, and seven (14.5 percent) had junior college or associate degrees (including three nurses). No one had less than a high school education.

Occupation

Occupations were just as varied as education. Fourteen (29.9 percent) indicated occupations within the health care field: There were two M.D.'s. five nurses, two mental health workers, and one each occupational therapist, physical therapist, respiratory therapist, dental hygienist, and radiology technician.

Two participants were certified massage therapists. Three were employed in the computer field, three were secretaries, three were homemakers. Five indicated jobs in administrative and management fields. One was a Catholic priest. The remainder (17) represented a variety of blue-collar positions, such as driver, counter salesperson, carpenter, mechanic, and food service worker.

Religious Preference

As indicated earlier, Reiki seems to cross all ethnic and cultural barriers. It is not confined to one or two religious persuasions. In the experimental group, twenty-three participants (47.9%) indicated a recognizable religious preference. Of these, six were Catholic, three were Buddhist, and two attend Unity churches. Surprisingly, two stated they were Jehovah's Witnesses, a group not often affiliated with healing groups. The remainder were Unitarian, Lutheran, Baptist, Protestant, Bahai, and Jewish (one each). Four did not name a denomination, but indicated "Christian."

Nine (18.8 percent) claimed no religious preference, while six (12.5 percent) indicated a "New Age" affiliation. The last ten (20.8 percent) had their own definitions of religion noting "God and me" (2), "universal" (3), "my own" (3), "Neopagan" (1), or "meditation" (1).

Excerpt from Significance

The interest in Reiki truly seems to cross all national, religious, and educational boundaries. It also seems indicative of Reiki's claim to not interfere with an individual's belief system or reference base....

Excerpts from Experiential Profile

Health and Health Habits

Participants were asked about their habits which related to health. It was believed that this group would be "health-conscious," and participate in activities which reflected this.

Participants were asked: Do you practice any of the following on a regular basis? Choices included: meditation, regular physical exercise, prayer, guided imagery, self-hypnosis, and any other as defined by the participant. The majority (42 = 87.5 percent) indicated that they did participate in these activities. The average response was 2.1 practices. A summary of the replies obtained follows.

SUMMARY OF HEALTH-RELATED PRACTICES

Practice	Number	Percent
Regular physical exercise	31	64.5%
Meditation	23	47.9%
Prayer	22	45.8%
Guided Imagery	13	27.0%
Self-Hypnosis	6	12.5%
Other		
Yoga	2	4.2%
Tai Chi	2	4.2%
QiGung	2	4.2%
Reasoning	1	2.0%
Course in Miracles	1	2.0%
Creative Imagery	1	2.0%
NeuroLinguistic Programming	1	2.0%
Affirmations	1	2.0%
Total Responses	106	
Responses per subject - mean	2.2	

Motivation

The research addressed the question: Why do people take Reiki? The researcher expected the primary reasons would be to use Reiki as a healing technique for others (as opposed to self-healing). However, both healing for others and personal growth were the most often cited. Self or personal healing was the next most frequent reason. See the following table.

SUMMARY OF REASONS FOR PARTICIPATING IN THE REIKI TRAINING

Reason	Number	Percent
Personal Growth	38	20.7%
Healing for Others	38	20.7%
Personal Healing	37	20.1%
Spiritual Growth	31	16.8%
Professional Growth	19	10.4%
Just Curious	15	8.2%
Other:		
Continuing Education credit for nurses	3	1.6%
"Alignment of purpose."	1	0.5%
"Want to see the change."	1	0.5%
"I just like it."	1	0.5%
Total	184	
Responses per subject - mean	3.8	

SUMMARY OF REACTIONS TO TREATMENTS

Emotional Reactions	Physical Reactions	Psychic Reactions	Energetic Reactions

clarity
self-love
peace
healing
balancing
calm
fullness
love
trust
safe and secure
spacy
smiling
released negative
  feelings
decrease stress
compassion
comfort
centered
harmony
	warmth or heat
	relaxation
	hot flushed face
	headache
	backache
	hot hands
	pressure in hands
	hunger
	cold
	decreased pain
		seeing lights
		seeing colors
		visual images
		throbbing 3rd eye
		  and hands
		unseen hands on body
			pulsations
			rise and fall of energy flow
			shifting energy
			tingling
			energy released through feet
			electricity

SUMMARY OF REACTIONS TO ATTUNEMENTS

Emotional Reactions	Physical Reactions	Psychic Reactions	Energetic Reactions

security
mellow
fear of "not getting it"
calm
relaxed
peace
centered
balanced
unity, oneness
settling
increased feelings
self-love
clarity of mind
reinforcement of mission
love
nurturing
freedom
contentment
joy
increased awareness
	heat in hands
	heat in head
	generalized warmth
	tingling hands
	tingling head
	hands moving and opening
	face flushing
	increased smell
	headache
	sounds
	breeze
	backache
	straight back
	dizzy, lightheaded
	giggling
		seeing colors
		seeing purple halo
		visualizations
		seeing lights
		seeing spirit
		  guides
		separation from
		  body
		crown chakra
		  activity
		3rd eye activity
		opening heart
		time travel
		designing jewelry
		  in the mind
		pulling force
		  within body
			energy flowing
			vibrations

Appendix B

A STUDY OF THE RELAXATION RESPONSE AND SUPPORT FOR HEALING THROUGH THE USUI SYSTEM OF NATURAL HEALING

Undergraduate Research
The Evergreen State College, Olympia, Washington
by
Penny L. Devine, Reiki Master

ABSTRACT

Definition of the Term "REIKI"

This study is based on work using the original "Usui System of Natural Healing," which introduced the term "Reiki" in the world.

The initiations, precepts, classes, and treatment guidelines are those passed on through the lineage of the Grand Masters in the Usui System, and are those supported and directed by The Reiki Alliance, the global association of Masters in The Usui System of Natural Healing. The lineage of the primary participants of this study are fifth and sixth generation initiates through Dr. Mikao Usui, Dr. Chujiro Hayashi, Rev. Hawayo Takata, Phyllis Lei Furumoto, and Penny L. Devine.

There are several other energy systems which have begun to use the title "Reiki," defined loosely to mean the use of "Universal Life Energy" in whatever vibrational system they may have developed. Any assumptions as to other systems producing the same results as shown in this study would need to be verified in the future by the practitioners of those other systems, and cannot be assumed.

Purpose
Many of today's maladies appear to be linked to a high level of stress in the patient's life. Many reports of Reiki's benefits indicate more than the simple relief of stress. The effects reported range from nearly-instantaneous healings of burns and other acute symptoms to the shrinking of tumors, alleviation of side effects of radiation and chemotherapy, and other significant healing experiences. Most of these reports are not easily documentable and could be partially credited to the use of other supportive measures in addition to the Reiki. The purpose of this study is to document some effects of Reiki on the stress release response of the participants, as measured by vital signs, biofeedback, and self-reports.

Procedures
All participants completed "The Change Scale," by Rahe and Holme (a questionnaire designed to evaluate the participant's potential for illness or accident), a participant profile (designed to record basic life style/health choices in the areas of diet, exercise, stress levels, health care practices—wholistic and allopathic, etc.), and a self-evaluation of perceptions of physical, mental, emotional and spiritual responses to class.

Vital signs (blood pressure, heart rate, temperature and respiration) were taken on Reiki students at the beginning and end of the first day of class, at the end of the class, and one week after completion of class. Additionally, clients were tested with biofeedback before and during a Reiki treatment.

A control group with no exposure to Reiki had vital signs taken at corresponding time.

Excerpts from Demographics, Reiki Participants

Sex , Age and Marital Status:
> Males - 7 , Females - 18
> Age - 2 in 20s, 6 in 30s, 10 in 40s, 3 in 50s, 1 was 69
> Married - 9, Unmarried (single, separated, divorced or widowed) - 13

Education:
> High school degrees - 4
> Undergraduate college students - 3
> PhD degrees - 2
> Bachelors degree - 16

Occupation:
> Students, a researcher, a psychic counselor, a high school counselor, a secretary, a state employee, an association executive, a lobbyist, a mother, a firefighter, a computer systems analyst, 2 accountants, a computer operator and a telephone technician.

Physical conditions:
> Heart block, birth defect, thyroid imbalance, colitis

Stress levels as reported on "The Change Scale":
> 56, 70, 86, 109, 127, 142, 170, 228, 337, 416
> average of 174

Excerpts from Demographics, Control Group

Sex, Age, and Marital Status:
> All unmarried females (single, separated, divorced or widowed)

Education:
> All students of The Evergreen State College enrolled in Human Health and Behavior

Occupation:
> Students, plus a photo lab printer, a plans examiner, 2 assistant managers and a cafe worker

Physical conditions:
> Cancer in remission, diabetes

Stress levels as reported on "The Change Scale":
> 0, 0, 60, 92, 114, 134, 208, 216, 248, 259, 437
> average of 161

Observations and Conclusions

I. THERE WAS OBVIOUS, IMMEDIATE GRAPH CONFIRMATION OF THE THERAPIST'S PERCEPTIONS OF ENERGY FLUCTUATIONS.

One of the first things Reiki students learn is that they will begin to feel the different frequencies and intensities in their hands as the energy ebbs and flows during treatment. This was dramatically presented as I watched the biofeedback graph during a treatment. I would apply my hands, the energy would begin to flow, the graph would begin to show an immediate increase in extremity temperature, which indicates deepening levels of relaxation. As the energy began to subside in my hands, the graph would level off at the acquired level of heat/relaxation.

We are taught that when this energy subsides it is telling us it is time to move our hands. So I would gently apply my hands to the next position and wait to feel the energy begin to flow. As the energy began to flow again, the graph again would begin a slow, steady rate of increase of heat/relaxation until the energy again began to wane.

This pattern was repeated over and over again and would continue until the person would reach his or her deepest level of relaxation.

II. IMMEDIATE CONFIRMATION OF LOSS OF CONSCIOUSNESS WAS ALSO EASILY OBSERVED ON THE GRAPH SCREEN.

When the client would move into an altered state of consciousness (i.e. asleep, or deeply meditating) the blood flow would switch from the extremities to the major organs and the extremity temperature would make an immediate and constant drop.

III. CONFIRMATION OF EMOTIONAL RESPONSE TO TREATMENT

During Reiki the client many times finds emotional or mental attitudes and situations correlate with the parts of the body treated. In these situations, many times the client will become aware of body metaphors that are direct descriptions of mental situations.

When these situations arose, the graph would also make an immediate dip, indicating the lack of relaxation and the tenseness the situation brings up in mind and body. After the crisis of the mental situation passed, the client would again move into the deeply relaxed state and the hand temperature would again begin its slow and steady rise.

IV. BIOFEEDBACK RELAXATION RESPONSE READINGS

While giving instructions on the use of his equipment, Mr. Grant indicated that during his years of using the biofeedback equipment he had seen the extremity[1] relaxation temperature reach 94.4 degrees[2] in only one situation, and that had been under the influence of drugs.

During our research, the warming trends were obvious in that they surpassed the above norms as a whole. All but three participants reached or excelled the relaxed norm[3] temperature; and of those who reached the relaxed norm, only two failed to meet or pass the 94.4 degree mark (12 met or surpassed). Both of these participants, however, had a marked increase in their temperature. One rose 24 degrees to reach 93.21 and the other rose 14.46 degrees to reach 91.24. Neither of these in my opinion would be a negative statistic in this study.

Mr. Grant indicated that the EMG muscle relaxation responses he observed on the data obtained through the neck muscle tension probe showed a marked level of relaxation as well. With one exception, where the tenseness increased considerably during the session, all muscle tension readings indicated the participants met the low relaxed norm reading of 1.6 to 3.0[4] most of whom (12 out of 17) surpassed this norm in an average time of 14 minutes.

V. VITAL STATISTICS RESPONSE OBSERVATIONS

Betty Bews observed that those participants in the vital statistics portion of the study with little stress in their lives would not be expected to and did not show large responses. In the control group, there was less stress as a whole in their lives and nearly all use drugs, both prescription and recreational.

In order to make a more accurate assessment we would have needed to know what drugs, at what strengths and at what frequencies were being taken by the participants in order to determine the effect of this variable on the results.

Even with the above considerations there was a significant lowering of all four vital signs during the Reiki class, even though the response was different in each participant. The base line of only four days does not show the more vast changes that the figures from one week later show.

VI. IRREGULAR PEAKS OF STRESS INDICATED ON GRAPHS

It is difficult to read the relaxation graphs unless you bear in mind that any time the client moved his or her head, turned over, or simply adjusted the head position, the muscle stress indicator would rise considerably and then return to the norm. This peak and fall is readily apparent on nearly all of the muscle relaxation graphs.

It is important for your eye to follow the general rise and fall of the tension in the muscle and ignore the short term peaks which indicate head motion.

---

[1]   Extremity Relaxation Temperature is taken on the dominant hand on the underside middle finger at first joint.
[2]   88–92 degrees is the average temperature range at the relaxed norm.
[3]   "The relaxed norm" state, which means generally composed in a reclining position or lying for at least 5 minutes.
[4]   1.6 to 3.0 is the relaxed norm value range for EMG readings.

Appendix C

AURA SKETCHES

On the following pages are sketches, done both before and after attunements, in First Degree Reiki and Second Degree Reiki classes.The sketches were done by some of our Reiki therapists who have the ability to see auras, better known as clairvoyants. The sketches were done with artists pastels and colored pencils on slightly textured white paper.

I wish to thank all of our students for taking part in the project. I just wish we could have put all of their beautiful pictures into the book.

A very special thanks, and much Reiki love, goes to our wonderful clairvoyants:

Paula Williams
Liz Howell-Kauffman
Pat Hodge
Isreal Wareham
Cindy Mikiel
Julie Edul
Fran Robins
Carol Nunez

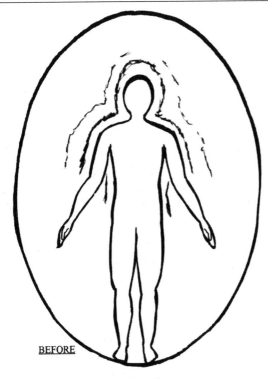

BEFORE

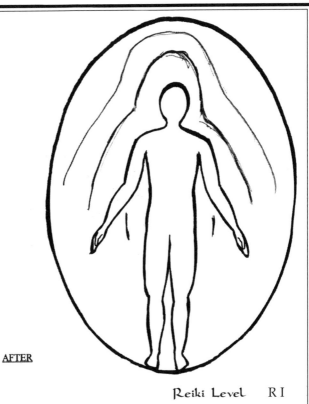

AFTER

Client's Name   Paul

Reiki Level   R I

Clairvoyant's Name   Liz Howell Kauffman

Date   10-20-95

Comments   Very interesting because he had a strong aura before, but after - WOW ! Much clearer and stronger

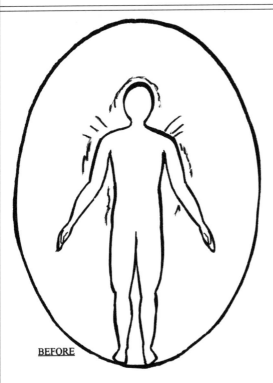

BEFORE

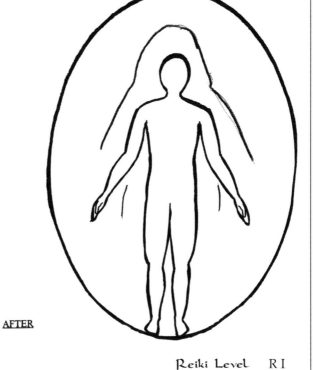

AFTER

Client's Name   Riki

Reiki Level   R I

Clairvoyant's Name   Liz Howell Kauffman

Date   10-20-95

Comments   Very soft, fluffy - lots of little leaks - a real giver - after the field is firm and clearer.

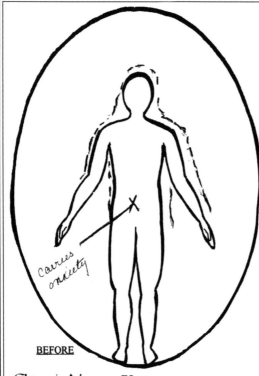

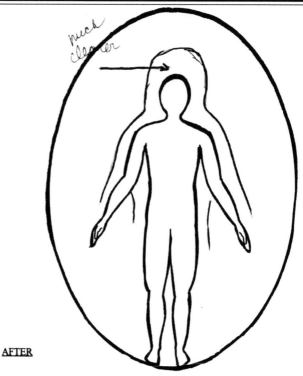

BEFORE

AFTER

Client's Name BJ

Reiki Level   R I

Clairvoyant's Name Liz Howell Kauffman

Date   10-20-95

Comments Before: aura pulled in tight on right side of body, bigger but dissipates on left. After: more balanced, stronger, clearer, appears to have had some releasing.

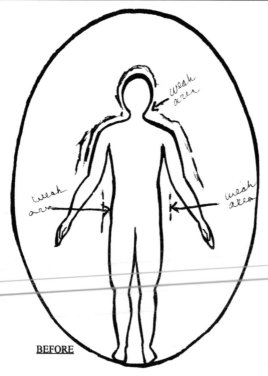

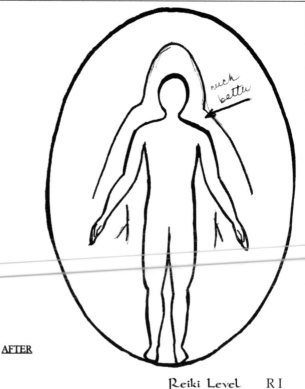

BEFORE

AFTER

Client's Name Don

Reiki Level   R I

Clairvoyant's Name Liz Howell Kauffman

Date   10-20-95

Comments Leaks were closed, aura bigger and clearer

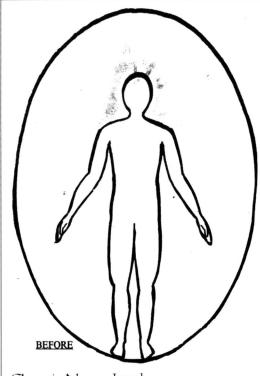
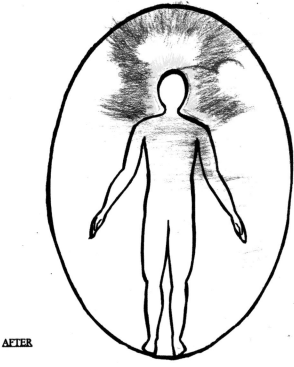

BEFORE

AFTER

Client's Name Isreal

Reiki Level R II

Clairvoyant's Name Carol

Date 11-12-95

Comments Blue attachment to guide, bright white light (symbolized by white with silver liner in front)

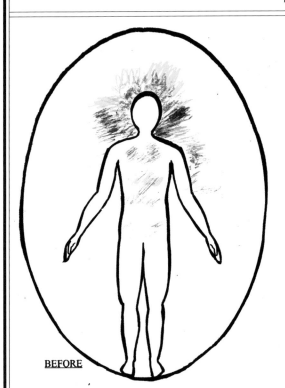
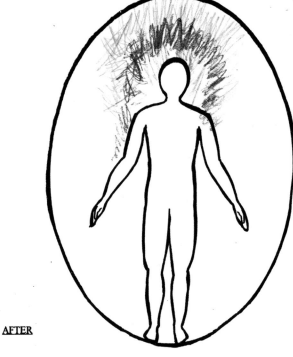

BEFORE

AFTER

Client's Name Michelle

Reiki Level R II

Clairvoyant's Name Fran Robins

Date 11-12-95

Comments

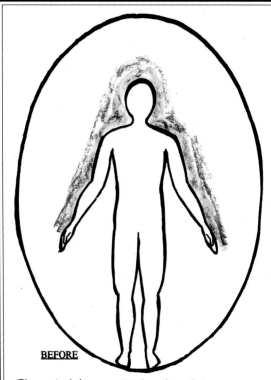
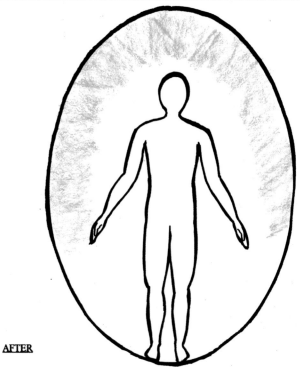

BEFORE

AFTER

Client's Name   Ricky (female)

Clairvoyant's Name   Anonymous

Date   10-20-95   Comments

Reiki Level   R I

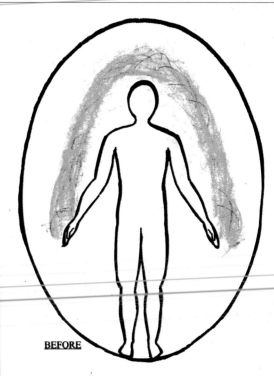
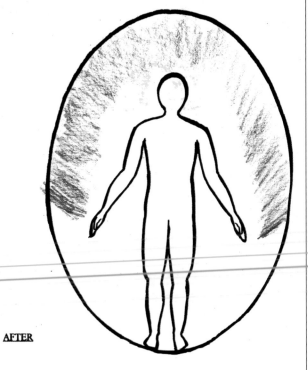

BEFORE

AFTER

Client's Name   Karen

Clairvoyant's Name   Anonymous

Date   10-20-95   Comments

Reiki Level   R I

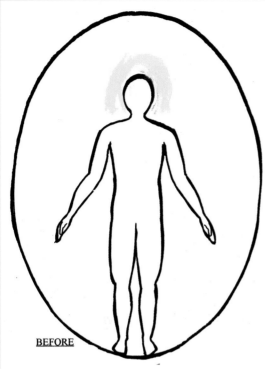
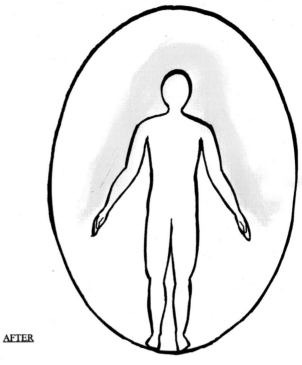

BEFORE

AFTER

Client's Name   Don

Reiki Level   R I

Clairvoyant's Name   Julie Edul

Date   10-20-95   Comments

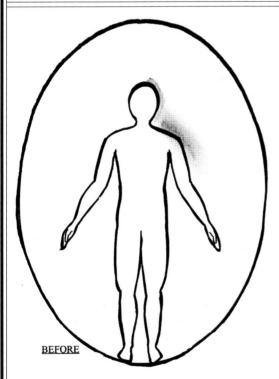
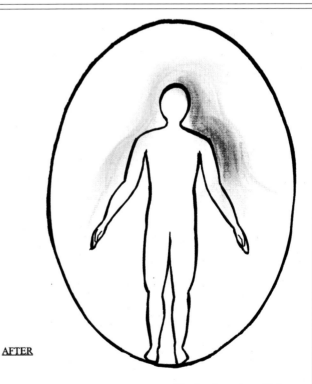

BEFORE

AFTER

Client's Name   Daniel

Reiki Level   R I

Clairvoyant's Name   Julie Edul

Date   10-20-95   Comments

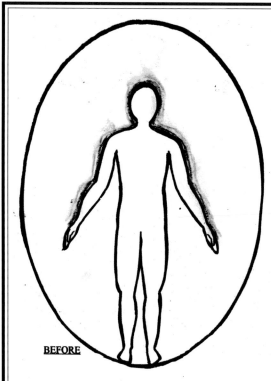

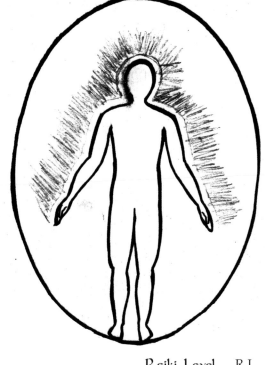

BEFORE

AFTER

Client's Name Ann

Reiki Level   R I

Clairvoyant's Name   Isreal

Date 11-10-95   Comments

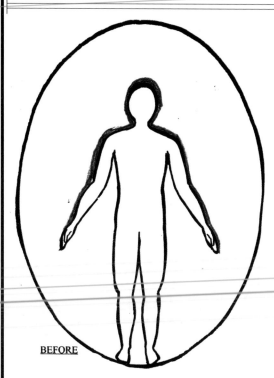

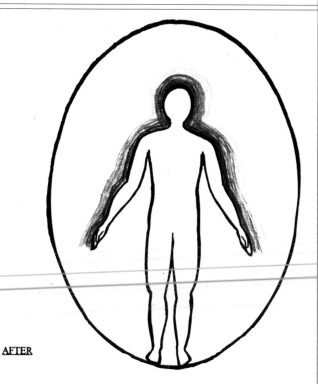

BEFORE

AFTER

Client's Name   America

Reiki Level   R I

Clairvoyant's Name   Isreal

Date   10-10-95   Comments

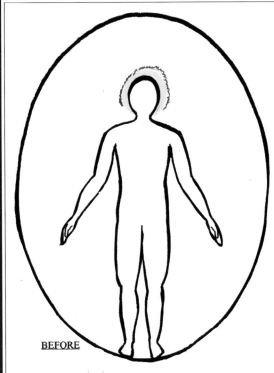

BEFORE

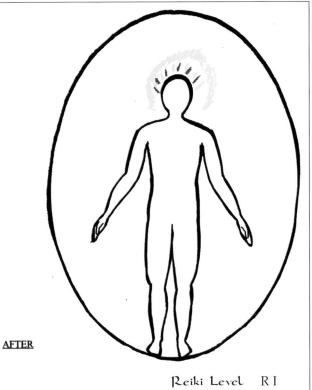

AFTER

Client's Name Don

Clairvoyant's Name Pat

Date 10-21-95

Reiki Level R I

Comments "Before" is Sat. AM (already has 1st two attunements) while Joyce is telling history of Reiki. "After" is after final attunements.

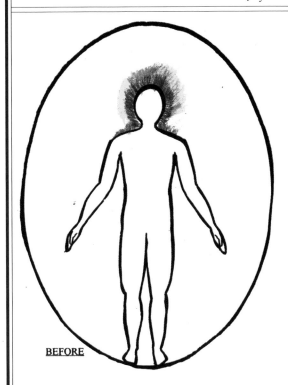

BEFORE

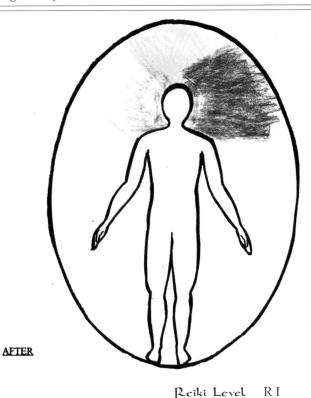

AFTER

Client's Name America

Clairvoyant's Name Cindy

Date 11-10-95

Reiki Level R I

Comments Gray at left on "after" sketch represents white light

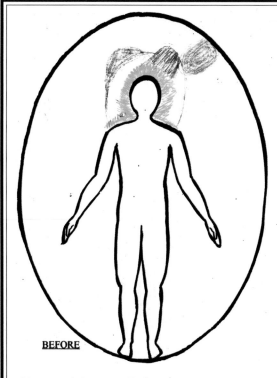 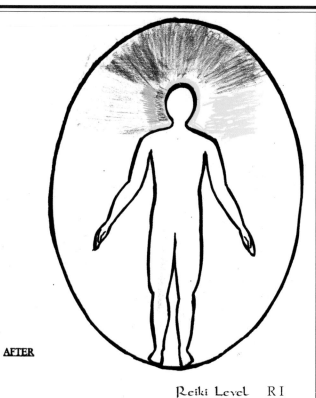

BEFORE **AFTER**

Client's Name   Delima   Reiki Level   R I

Clairvoyant's Name Cindy

Date   11-10-95   Comments   Right top, above head, was entity or guide. Gray at left
(after) is white light.

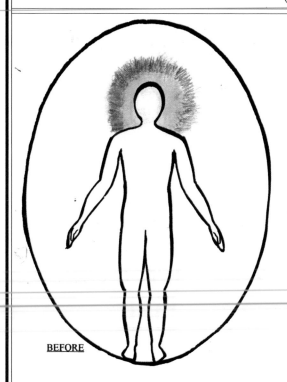 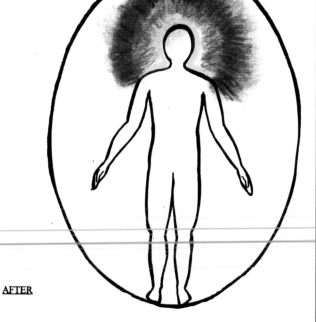

BEFORE **AFTER**

Client's Name   Anne   Reiki Level   R I

Clairvoyant's Name Cindy

Date   11-10-95   Comments

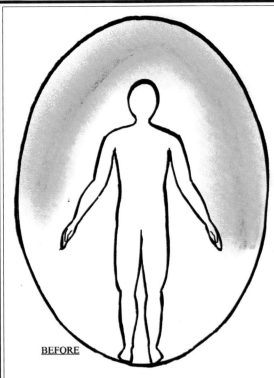
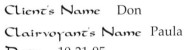

BEFORE

AFTER

Client's Name   Don

Clairvoyant's Name   Paula

Date   10-21-95   Comments

Reiki Level   R I

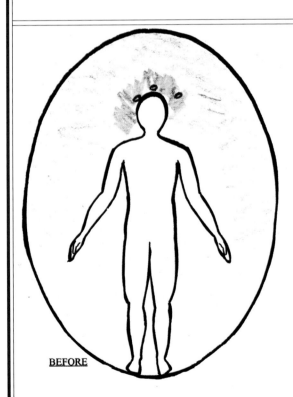
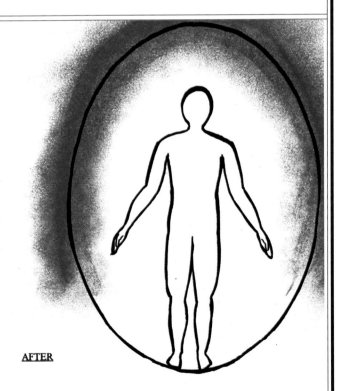

BEFORE

AFTER

Client's Name   John

Clairvoyant's Name   Paula

Date   10-21-95   Comments

Reiki Level   R I

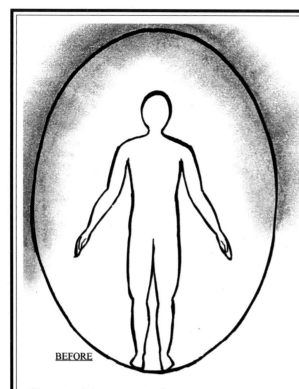
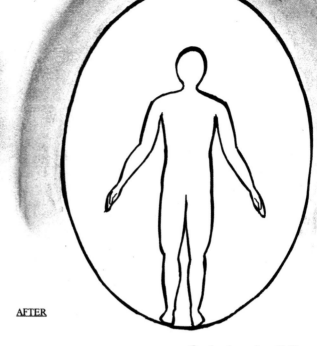

BEFORE

AFTER

Client's Name   Kathy

Reiki Level   R II

Clairvoyant's Name Paula

Date   10-22-95   Comments   Pale blue iridescent to pale lavender iridescent

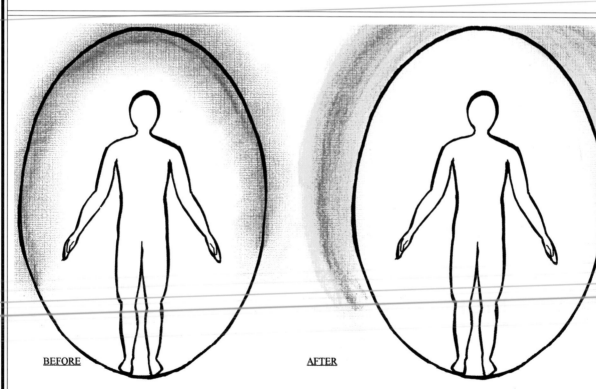

BEFORE

AFTER

Client's Name   Daniel

Reiki Level   R II

Clairvoyant's Name Paula

Date   10-22-95   Comments Final aura orange (iridescent) gold

Appendix D

BIBLE REFERENCES ON COLORS AND CRYSTALS (GEMSTONES)

The Complete Bible, J.M. Powis Smith, ed. Chicago, IL: University of Chicago Press, 1923.

The Book of Exodus, 28:4-22

The following are the vestments that they must make: a pouch, an apron, a robe, a tunic in checkered work, a turban, and a sash. They must make the sacred vestments for your brother Aaron and his sons, that he may serve as priest to me; and they must use gold, violet, purple, and scarlet material, and fine linen.

"They must make the apron of gold, violet, purple, and scarlet material, and fine twisted linen, in skilled work; it must have two shoulder-straps joined to it at the two ends, and thus be joined. The skilfully made girdle on it must be made like it, of one piece with it, of gold, violet, purple, and scarlet material, and fine twisted linen. You must then procure two onyx stones, and engrave on them the names of the Israelites, six of their names on the one stone, and the remaining six on the other stone, in the order of their origin; with seal engravings, the work of a jeweler, you must engrave the two stones with the various names of the Israelites, setting them in filigree work of gold; and you must fasten the two stones on the shoulder-straps of the apron, as memorial stones for the Israelites, and so Aaron shall carry their names on his shoulders in the presence of the LORD as a memorial.

"You must also make filigree objects of gold, and two chains of pure gold, making them of twisted material, of cordage-work, and you must fasten the corded chains to the filigree objects.

"Further, you must make an oracle pouch in skilled work; you must make it in the same way as the apron, making it of gold, violet, purple, and scarlet material, and fine twisted linen; it is to be square, and folded double, a span long, and a span wide; and you must insert in it a setting of stones, four rows of stones, the first row to be a row of carnelian, topaz, and emerald, the second row a ruby, a sapphire, and a crystal, the third row a jacinth, an agate, and an amethyst, and the fourth row a chrysolite, an onyx, and a jasper; they are to be inclosed with gold in their settings. The stones, corresponding to the names of the Israelites, are to be twelve in number, as their names are, each to be engraved like a seal with its proper name for the twelve tribes.

The Book of Exodus 39: 8-14

Then the pouch was made, the work of artists, like that of the apron, in gold, violet, purple, and scarlet material, and fine twisted linen; the pouch was square, being made double, a span long, and a span wide, folded double; and on it were set four rows of stones, the first row a row of carnelian, topaz, and emerald, the second row a ruby, a sapphire, and a crystal, the third row a jacinth, an agate, and an amethyst, and the fourth row a chrysolite, an onyx, and a jasper; they were inclosed in gold filigree in their settings. The stones, corresponding to the names of the Israelites, were twelve in number, as their names are, each engraved like a seal with its proper name for the twelve tribes.

Appendix E

ADDRESSES AND PHONE NUMBERS

REIKI CENTER OF LOS ANGELES
16161 Ventura Blvd., Suite 802
Encino, CA 91436
Phone: (818) 881-5959
Fax: (818) 881-1613
http://www.REIKI-CENTER.ORG
http://www.FENG-SHUI-DESIGNS.COM
Founder and Director: Joyce Morris, M.S., C.A.D.C., N.C.A.C. II, Reiki Master Teacher
Purpose: Education of the public about Reiki and a support organization for Reiki Center Therapists.

THE REIKI ALLIANCE
P.O. Box 41
Cataldo, ID 83810-1041
Phone: (208) 682-3535
FAX: 1-208-682-4848
Email: ReikiAlliance@compuserve.com
Executive Director: Connie Hoy
Purpose: An Alliance of Reiki Masters formed to support its members in teaching the Mikao Usui System of Reiki.

THE DEVINE REIKI GROWTH CENTER
Penny L. Devine, Reiki Master Teacher
2002 Capitol Way, South
Olympia, WA 98501
(306) 754-9750
Email: devineshire@worldnet.att.net

Bibliography

Achterberg, Jeanne, Barbara Dossey and Leslie Kolkmeier. *Rituals of Healing: Using Imagery for Health and Wellness.* New York: Bantam, 1994.

Amber, Ruben. *Color Therapy.* Santa Fe, NM: Aurora, 1983.

American Psychiatric Association. *Diagnostic and Statistical Manual of Mental Disorders, Third Edition.* Washington, DC: American Psychiatric Association, 1987.

Arnold, Larry E. and Sandra K. Nevius. *The Reiki Handbook.* 4th Edition. Harrisburg, PA: PSI Press, 1992.

Babbitt, Edwin. *The Principles of Light & Color.* Faber Birren, ed. Secaucus, NJ: Citadel Press, 1967.

Baginski, Bodo J. and Shalila Sharamon. *Reiki: Universal Life Energy.* Mendocino, CA: Life Rhythm, 1988.

Barnett, Libby, et al. *Reiki Energy Medicine: Bringing the Healing Touch into Home, Hospital, & Hospice.* (Rochester, VT: Inner Traditions, 1996).

Baum, Joseph. *The Beginner's Handbook of Dowsing.* New York: Crown, 1974.

Becker, Robert O., M. D. and Gary Selden. *The Body Electric.* New York: Quill Press, 1985.

Benson, Herbert, and Miriam Z. Klipper. *The Relaxation Response.* New York: Avon, 1976.

Bloch, Douglas. *Listening to Your Inner Voice.* Minneapolis, MN: CompCare, 1991.

———. *Words That Heal.* New York: Bantam, 1990.

Borysenko, Joan. *Minding the Body, Mending the Mind.* Reading, MA: Addison-Wesley, 1987.

Brennan, Barbara Ann. *Hands of Light.* New York: Bantam, 1991.

———. *Light Emerging: The Journey of Personal Healing.* New York: Bantam, 1993.

Brodeur, Paul. *Currents of Death.* New York: Simon & Schuster, 1989.

———. *The Great Power-Line Coverup.* New York: Little, Brown & Co., 1993.

Brown, Fran. *Living Reiki: Takata's Story.* Mendocino, CA: Life Rhythm, 1992.

Bruyère, Rosalyn. *Wheels of Light: A Study of the Chakras, Vol . I.* Sierra Madre, CA: Bon Productions, 1989.

Callahan, Peter. "A Healthy Room is a Leafy Room." *Omni Magazine.* September, 1993.

Carson, Richard D. *Taming Your Gremlin.* New York: Harper & Row, 1983.

Chinmoy, Sri. *Beyond Within.* Jamaica, NY: Agni Press, 1974.

Choa, Kok Sui. *Pranic Healing.* York Beach, ME: Samuel Weiser, 1990.

Chopra, Deepak. *Ageless Body, Timeless Mind.* New York: Harmony, 1993.

———. *Perfect Health.* New York: Harmony, 1993.

———. *Quantum Healing.* New York: Bantam, 1989.

Clark Linda. *The Ancient Art of Color Therapy.* Old Greenwich, CT: Devin-Adair Co., 1975.

"Cleaning Your Indoor Air: Mum's the Word." *New Age Journal.*

Complete Bible J. M. Powis Smith, ed. Chicago, IL: University of Chicago Press, 1923.

Cousins, Norman. *The Healing Heart.* New York: Avon, 1983.

———. *Anatomy of an Illness as Perceived by the Patient.* New York: Bantam, 1981.

Dadd, Debra Lynn. *Nontoxic, Natural and Earthwise.* Los Angeles: Jeremy P. Tarcher, 1990.

———. *The Nontoxic Home & Office.* Los Angeles: Jeremy P. Tarcher, 1992.

———. *The Nontoxic Home.* Los Angeles: Jeremy P. Tarcher, 1986.

Davies, Rodney. *Dowsing: the Art of Finding Hidden Things.* San Francisco: Thorsons, 1991.

Diamond, John. *Your Body Doesn't Lie.* New York: Warner Books, 1989.

Eos, Nancy. *Reiki and Medicine.* Laytonville, CA: White Feather, 1995.

Fetzler, William. *Creative Imagery.* New York: Simon & Schuster, 1989.

Gawain, Shakti. *Creative Visualization.* Mill Valley, CA: Nataraj, 1978.

———. *Living in the Light.* Mill Valley, CA: Nataraj Publishing, 1986.

Goleman, Daniel. "The Art of Meditation." Los Angeles, Audio Renaissance Tapes, 1989.

Haberly, Helen J. *Reiki: Hawayo Takata's Story.* Olney, MD: Archedigm Publications, 1990.

Haich, Elizabeth. *The Day with Yoga.* Santa Fe, NM: Aurora, 1987.

Halpern, Steven. "Spectrum Suite." San Anselmo, CA: Inner Peace Music.

Hay Louise. *You Can Heal Your Life.* Carson, CA: Hay House, 1984.

Hayward, Susan. *Begin it Now.* Hayward, CA: In-Tune Books, 1989.

———. *A Guide for the Advanced Soul.* New York: Little Brown, 1989.

Hornik, Susan. "How to Get that Extra Edge on Health and Wealth." *Smithsonian.* August, 1993.

Howell, Kelly. "Brain Sync" series. Santa Fe, NM: Brain Sync Corp.

Joy, Brugh. "Healing with Body Energy." Los Angeles, CA: Audio Renaissance Tapes, 1987.

Karp, Reba A. *Edgar Cayce Encyclopedia of Healing.* New York: Warner, 1988.

King, Serge. *Imagineering for Health.* Wheaton, IL: Quest Books, 1991.

Kreiger, Dolores. *Therapeutic Touch: How to Use Your Hands to Help or to Heal.* New York: Simon & Schuster, 1979.

Krippner, Stanley and Daniel Rubin, eds. *The Kirlian Aura: Photographing the Galaxies of Life.* Garden City, NY: Doubleday, 1974.

Lao Tsu. *Tao Te Ching.* Gia-fu Feng and Jane English, eds. New York: Random House, 1972.

Lieberman, Joseph. *Light: The Medicine of the Future.* Santa Fe, NM: Bear & Co., 1991.

Lugenbeel, Barbara D. *Virginia Samdahl: Reiki Master Healer.* Norfolk, VA: Grunwald and Radcliff, 1984.

McGarey, William. *The Edgar Cayce Remedies.* New York: Bantam, 1983.

Mengle, Kathy. *Tools for Healing: Working toward Harmony and Balance.* Marina Del Rey, CA: DeVorss & Company, 1987.

Mermet, Abbé, *Principles and Practice of Radiesthesia.* Rockport, MA: Element, 1990.

Morris, Joyce J. "Getting in Touch With Your Higher Self." Encino, CA: Reiki, 1990.

———. "Healing I—Color Breathing and Affirmations." Encino, CA: Reiki, 1990.

———. "Healing II—Water Purification." Encino, CA: Reiki, 1991.

Morris, William. "Helios Attunements." Santa Monica, CA: Helios, 1988.

———. "Helios Rising." Santa Monica, CA: Helios, 1984.

Oslie, Pamela. *Life Colors.* Novato, CA: New World Library, 1991.

Ott, John N. *Health and Light.* Old Greenwich, CT: Devin-Adair Co., 1973.

———. *Light, Radiation & You: How to Stay Healthy.* Old Greenwich, CT: Devin-Adair Co., 1985.

Ponder, Catherine. *Open Your Mind to Prosperity.* Marina Del Ray, CA: DeVorss & Company, 1971.

———. *The Dynamic Laws of Healing.* Marina Del Ray, CA: DeVorss & Company, 1966.

———. *The Healing Secrets of the Ages.* Marina Del Ray, CA: DeVorss & Company, 1985.

———. *The Prospering Power of Love.* Marina Del Ray, CA: DeVorss & Company, 1966.

Puryear, Herbert. *The Edgar Cayce Primer.* New York: Bantam, 1982.

Raphaell, Katrina. *Crystal Enlightenment.* Sante Fe, NM: Aurora, 1985.

———. *Crystal Healing.* Santa Fe, NM: Aurora, 1987.

Rossbach, Sarah. *Feng Shui: The Chinese Art of Placement.* London and New York: Arkana, 1991.

———. *Interior Design with Feng Shui.* London and New York: Arkana, 1991.

Seigel, Bernie S. *Peace, Love & Healing.* New York: HarperCollins, 1989.

———. *Love, Medicine & Miracles.* New York: HarperCollins, 1985.

Shinn, Florence Scovel. *The Wisdom of Florence Scovel Shinn.* New York: Simon & Schuster, 1989.

Silbey, Uma. *The Complete Crystal Guidebook.* San Francisco: U-Read Publications, 1987.

Smyth, Angela. *Seasonal Affective Disorder.* London: Thorsons, 1990.

Stewart, Judy-Carol. *The Reiki Touch.* Houston, TX: 1988.

Sugerman, Ellen. *Warning: The Electricity Around You May Be Hazardous to Your Health.* New York: Simon & Schuster, 1998.

Von Rohr, Ingrid S. *Harmony is the Healer.* Rockport, MA: Element, 1992.

Walker, Dael. *The Crystal Healing Handbook.* Pacheco, CA: The Crystal Co., 1988.

Weil, Andrew. *Natural Health, Natural Medicine.* Boston: Houghton Mifflin, 1990.

Wetzel, Wendy S. *Reiki Healing: Physiologic Perspective and Implications for Nursing.* Masters Thesis, Sonoma State University, Sonoma, CA, 1988.

Yogananda, Paramahansa. *Man's Eternal Quest.* Los Angeles, CA: Self-Realization Fellowship, 1975.

Zdenek, Marilee. *Inventing the Future: Advances in Imagery That Can Change Your Life.* New York: McGraw-Hill, 1987.

Seminar Information

At the Reiki Seminar, Master/Trainer Joyce Morris transformed me into a human antenna to receive broadcasts of universal energy. After a two-day training, I was a certified Reiki practitioner; I could channel energy—with no additional training required—for the rest of my life, merely by putting my hands on myself, another human, or any living thing.

—Robert Andrews
Whole Life Times/June 1985

I currently teach both Reiki and Feng Shui seminars on a regular basis throughout California, Colorado, and the Berkshires in New England. I am available to teach seminars in other areas as the students appear. My First Degree Reiki class is usually held on Friday evening and all day Saturday, for a total of 13 hours. Second Degree is an all-day class, usually held on a Sunday. Feng Shui classes are taught as either a one-day class, or as one or more evening sessions.

Continuing education hours are available for my classes in California for both nurses and alcohol & drug counselors. Many other professional organizations and other states have also honored these classes for professional credit.

I am available to present lectures and classes at both Expos and conferences as they fit into my current teaching schedule. Everything I teach—Reiki, Feng Shui, Guided Visualization, Wholistic Stress Management—I consider to be tools for transformation.

For current seminar information:

- call 1-818-881-5959
- or write to me at 16161 Ventura Blvd. # 802, Encino, CA 91436
- or e-mail me at http://www.REIKI-CENTER.org

I hope to meet you soon.

In Love and Light,

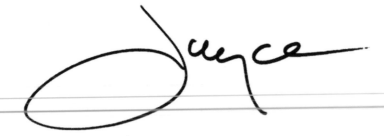

REIKI 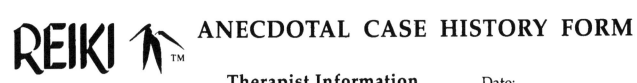 ANECDOTAL CASE HISTORY FORM

Therapist Information

Date: _____

Therapist's Name: _____
　　　　　　　　　　Last　　　　　　　　First　　　　　　　Middle

Address: _____
　　　　　Street　　　　　　　　City　　　　　State & Zip

Phone Number: Home _____ Work _____

Education: High School ____ College Degree ____ Post-Graduate ____ Other _____

Certification/License: MD ☐ DC ☐ LcA ☐ OMD ☐ MFCC ☐ Psychologist ☐
RN ☐ LVN ☐ CAC/CADC ☐ Mass.Ther. ☐ Minister ☐ Other _____

Therapist Reiki Level (with date): RI _____ RII _____ R3A _____ R3B _____

Trained by Reiki Master _____

Professional Affiliation: Reiki Alliance ☐ AIRA ☐ TRT ☐ Other _____

Client Information

Client's Name: _____
　　　　　　　Last　　　　　　　First　　　　　　Middle

Check here if Name is not to be used ☐

If Open to personal contact, please give:

Phone Number: _____

Address: _____

_____

Age: _____ Sex: _____ Marital Status: _____

Presenting Problem (include the length/duration of the problem, cause of problem, age/time problem began, allergies, medications used):

_____

_____

_____

_____

_____

_____

Medical Confirmation

Doctor's Name: _____

Address: _____

Phone Number: _____

Description of X-Ray or other Physical "before/after" confirmation data: _____

_____

_____

_____

Medical Treatment (past and current as pertains to current problem): _____

_____

_____

_____

Reiki Treatment

Date of 1st treatment, length and type (hands-on or absentee):

Dates of further treatments, length and type (hands on or absentee). Compare level of the problem, disability or dysfunction both before and after Reiki treatments:

Date	Length	Hands On	Absentee	Before	After

Index

A

A.A.. *See* Alcoholics Anonymous
A.L.S. 124
abscess 123, 126, 128
accidents 123
acne 124
acupressure 124
acupuncture 124
addictions 124, 126, 128, 134, 136
adrenals 123, 124
affirmations 58
aging 124
AIDS 67, 124, 132
Alcoholics Anonymous 60, 61. *See also* AA
alcoholism 66, 67
allergies 124, 125, 129
Alzheimer's 124
American International Reiki Association 29
anemia 124, 125
anorexia nervosa 124
anxiety 124
apprenticeship 11
ARC 125
arms 125, 129, 130
arthritis 10, 125, 126, 130, 135
asthma 71, 125
attunements 43, 44, 73, 83, 143
auras (auric fields) 47, 66, 73, 74, 75, 80, 149
auto-immune system disorders 125

B

backaches 125
baldness 125, 130
bed wetting 125
bee stings 125, 132
beggar 11
Beggar City 31
Bell's Palsy 125
Bible 167
biofeedback 72, 146, 147
bipolar 133
birthing 137
bleeding 125, 127
blisters 126

blood pressure 71, 72, 126
blood purification 124
Blood Purifier 63
blood replenisher 124
boils 126
brain injury 126, 130
breasts 126
breathing 47, 55, 59
broken bones 65, 69, 123, 126, 130
bronchitis 126
bulimia 126
burns 126, 137
bursitis 68, 126

C

calluses 126
cancer 68, 69, 126, 132
candida albicans 126
candle meditation 57
carbuncle 126
carpal tunnel 126
cataracts 66
cause and effect 62
Cayce, Edgar 56
cerebral palsy 126
chakra 47, 78, 85, 87, 91, 93, 97, 99, 101, 103, 105, 107, 109, 111, 113
chanting 57
chemotherapy 67, 68, 69, 126
Chi 81
childbirth 127, 135
Chinese Art of Placement 82
chiropractic 127
chronic fatigue syndrome 66, 127, 132
circulation 127, 138
cirrhosis 127
clairvoyance 74
colds 127, 130, 132, 135
colic 127
color 77, 78, 161
color breathing 60
coma 127
compulsive overeating 127
congenital defects 127

constipation 127
continuing education hours 168
corns 126
coughs 127
cramps 127
crystals 78, 80, 167
cuts 127
cystic fibrosis 127
cystitis 128
cysts 128

D
deafness 128
death 128, 137
dental 128, 130, 133, 135
depression 128
detoxification 55, 56, 58, 63, 124
Devine, Penny 72, 145, 163
Devine Reiki Growth Center 163
diabetes 128
dialysis 66, 128
diarrhea 128, 130
digestive disorders 128, 132
diverticulosis 128
dizziness 128
dowsing 73
dream recall 128
dropped foot 128
drug addictions 128

E
ears 128, 129
edema 129
electromagnetic fields 72, 73, 81
emotional disorders 128, 129, 133, 134, 135, 136, 137
emphysema 66, 67, 129
empowerment 65, 68
endometriosis 67
endorphins 134
energy 81, 129
energy, rise and fall of 47
enlightenment 137
environmental pollutants 80
environments, healing 57, 77
epilepsy 129
Epstein-Barr virus 67, 129, 132
equilibrium 128, 129
etheric 65, 73
ethics 39
eyes 69, 126, 129, 130

F
fasting 129

fatigue 129
feet 125, 129
Feng Shui 81, 168
fever 129
fibromyalgia syndrome 129
First Degree 43, 73
Five Principles of Reiki 11, 31, 32, *See also* Principles of Reiki
flu 130
food 130
food poisoning 130
fractures 130
free will 1, 53, 65
frostbite 130
Furumoto, Phyllis Lei 29

G
gall bladder 67, 130
gallstones 130
gas 130
gemstones 80, 161
glaucoma 130
gout 130
Graves Disease 125
grounding 130
guided visualization 58, 59, 168
gum problems 128, 130, 133
gums 135

H
hair 130
hand positions 83
hands 125, 130
hangover 130
Hayashi, Dr. Chujiro 12, 23, 29, 53
head injuries 130
headache, tension 130, 131, 133
healing crisis 55, 56
healing environments 77
health care, preventive 135
heart attack 131
heartburn 131
hematocrit 71, 139
hematoma 131
hemoglobin 71, 139
hemophilia 131
hemorrhage 131
hemorrhoids 131
hepatitis 131
hernia 131
hernia, hiatal 131
herpes 131
hiccups 131

high blood pressure 131
HIV+ 131, 132
homeopathy 131
hypertension 131
hypnosis 132, 134
hypoglycemia 132

I
immune system disorders 125, 126, 127, 129, 131, 132, 133
impotence 132
indigestion 132
infections 132
influenza 132
initiation 29, 44, 45, 73
initiation, Reiki 3
insect bites 132
insomnia 132
insulin 71

J
jaundice 132
joints 1

K
Karma (karmic) 1, 3, 61, 62, 65
kidney stone 67
kirlian photography 72

L
laryngitis 132
Law of Opposites 121
learning 132
legal 51
legs 125, 132
licenses 51
life style changes 61
light 77
light bearers 62
liver 131, 132
Lou Gehrig's Disease 66, 124
lupus 125, 132

M
manic-depressive 133
massage 133
master level 44
measles 133
meditation 57, 133
memory 132, 133
menopause 133
menopause, male 133
menstrual problems 127, 133, 135

mid-life crisis 133
migraine 130, 133
miracles 10, 65, 123
moles 133
Morris, William, O.M.D. 83, 121
motion sickness 133
Mount Kurama-yama 9
multiple sclerosis 133
mumps 134
muscular dystrophy 134

N
NASA 79, 80
nasal polyps 134
nausea 134
negative ions 80
nervousness 134
nosebleed 134

O
obesity 127, 134
organ clock 121
oriental medicine 83
Ott, Dr. John 77
ovarian cysts 67
overeating 134

P
pacing and leading 47
pain 134
paralysis 134
Parkinson's disease 134
past life recall 134
personal transformation 41
phobias 135
plants 79
pleurisy 135
PMS 135
pneumonia 135
pollution 79
Ponder, Catherine 62
positive thought 58
post traumatic stress disorder 68
prayer 56
pregnancy 135
premenstrual syndrome 135
principles 31
    See also Five Principles of Reiki
prosperity 37, 62
prostate 135
psoriasis 66, 137
psychomatic illness 135
PTSD See post traumatic stress disorder

purification 55, 59
pyorrhea 135

Q
quadriplegic 68
quick picker-upper 129

R
radiation 135
rage 65
rash 135
Ray, Barbara Weber 29
reflexology 135
Reiki Alliance 29, 163
Reiki Center 41, 163
reiki slaw 63, 124
reincarnation 1
relationship 66
relaxation 135
relaxation response 145
research 71, 139, 145
retina, detached 67, 128
rheumatism 135
rise and fall of energy 47

S
sacred ceremonies 31
SAD. *See* seasonal affective disorder
Samdahl, Virginia 13, 15, 27, 29
scars 135
schizophrenia 67, 136
sciatic nerve 136
scleroderma 136
seasonal affective disorder 77
second degree 44, 62, 63, 74, 123
senility 136
sexual problems 136
sexually transmitted diseases 136
shingles 136
shock 136
sick office syndrome 80
sickle-cell anemia 136
sinus 136
sleep apnea 136
sleep disorders 132, 136
smoking 136
snake bite 136
SOS. *See* sick office syndrome
sound 79, 80
spleen 123, 124, 126, 128, 134

sprain 137
stress management and reduction 15, 135, 137, 145
stress release response 72
stroke 137
stuttering 137
suicidal 67
sunburn 137
surgery 65, 67, 68, 137
sutras 9, 10

T
tachycardia 137
Takata, Madam Hawayo 12, 15, 25, 29, 48, 55, 77, 123
team treatments 51
Tempero-Mandibular Joint Dysfunction 137
temptations 53
tendinitis 126, 137
tenfold 62
tennis elbow 137
therapeutic touch 71, 139
third degree 44
thyroid 71, 137
tic douloureux 139
tinnitus 139
TMJ *See* Tempero-Mandibular Joint Dysfunction
tonsillitis 137
toxins 49, 131
transformation 43, 55, 57, 60, 62, 168
transformation tools 55
transition 128, 137
tumors 66, 69, 126, 138
Twelve Step 60, 61, 124

U
ulcers 138
Universal Life Energy 3, 7, 9
Usui, Dr. Mikao 3, 9, 10, 11, 21, 31, 34

V
vaginitis 138
varicose veins 138
venereal disease 138
vibratory energy 77, 78, 79
vomiting 138

W
warts 133
whiplash 138
White Light Meditation 58

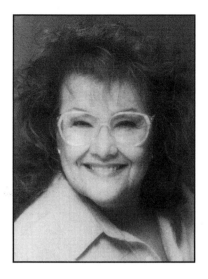

Joyce J. Morris, M.S., C.A.D.C., N.C.A.C. II
Reiki Master Teacher

Joyce Morris is Director of the Reiki Center of Los Angeles, a Certified Alcohol and Drug Counselor, a Certified Reality Therapist and a well known lecturer and teacher throughout the United States. She specializes in Reiki, Wholistic Stress Management, Guided Visualization and Feng Shui. Joyce has been on numerous TV and radio programs, and is a frequent presenter at state and national conferences.

Joyce has a B.S. from Purdue University, in Indiana, and a M.S. from Oklahoma State University. She is a member of the Alliance of Reiki Masters, the California and National Associations of Alcohol and Drug Abuse Counselors, and is also a California Certified Interior Designer. Joyce has an extensive metaphysical background and is interested in the effects pf the environment on health, homeopathy, acupressure, meditation, guided imagery and Feng Shui. In addition to *Reiki Hands that Heal*, Morris has produced guided visualization tapes for healing and spiritual growth.

She is a popular lecturer and runs seminars coast to coast. If you want more information about seminar locations, book signings, or private sessions, please contact the author at 818-881-5959, or write her at 16161 Ventura Blvd. # 802, Encino, CA 91436.

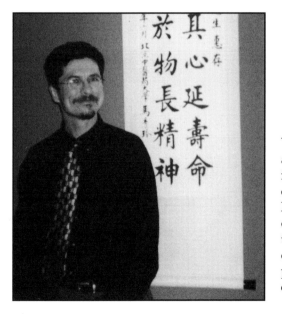

William R. Morris,
Lic. Ac., M. Ac., O.M.D.
Reiki Master Teacher

William Morris is Joyce's son, a noted teacher and published author specializing in cutting edge technology and treatment in the field of Oriental and Energy Medicine. He is a graduate of Emperor's College of Traditional Oriental Medicine in Santa Monica, CA, and Samra University also in Santa Monica. His doctoral and post doctoral work is in the traditional and contemporary modalities. He has taught at Williams College and developed a two year herbal medicine program qualifying acupuncturists for National Boards. William is the Academic Dean of Emperor's College of Traditional Oriental Medicine.